# SEX CELLS

# SEX CELLS

## THE FIGHT TO OVERCOME BIAS AND DISCRIMINATION IN WOMEN'S HEALTHCARE

Phyllis E. Greenberger, MSW
With Kalia Doner

MAYO CLINIC PRESS

MAYO CLINIC PRESS
200 First St. SW
Rochester, MN 55905
mcpress.mayoclinic.org

The information in this book is true and complete to the best of our knowledge. This book is intended as an informative guide for those wishing to learn more about health issues. It is not intended to replace, countermand or conflict with advice given to you by your own physician. The ultimate decision concerning your care should be made between you and your doctor. Information in this book is offered with no guarantees. The author and publisher disclaim all liability in connection with the use of this book. The views expressed are the author's personal views, and do not necessarily reflect the policy or position of Mayo Clinic.

To stay informed about Mayo Clinic Press, please subscribe to our free e-newsletter at mcpress.mayoclinic.org or follow us on social media.

For bulk sales to employers, member groups and health-related companies, contact Mayo Clinic at SpecialSalesMayoBooks@mayo.edu.

Proceeds from the sale of every book benefit important medical research and education at Mayo Clinic.

Cover design by Henry Sene Yee

Cover art by tru3_art / shutterstock.com

Library of Congress Control Number: 2023034456

ISBN: 979-8-88770-020-5 hardcover
ISBN: 979-8-88770-021-2 ebook

Printed in China
First edition: 2024

# CONTENTS

*In loving memory of my husband, Robert*

## PART 1

# Lead, Follow or Get Out of the Way

have been working in the field of biological sex differences for more than 30 years, first as the CEO and president of the Society for Women's Health Research and now as the senior vice president of Science and Health Policy for HealthyWomen. Despite the increased awareness of sex differences that has emerged lately, I am still struck by how often there is a lack of understanding about this topic, even among medical professionals. After all, it's fundamental: males and females are different biologically. What's more, those differences impact everything we know about how to diagnose and treat diseases—or they *should* impact everything we know about how to diagnose and treat diseases. The idea that our biological sex impacts our health seems like such a simple concept. Unfortunately, it has proven to be anything but.

First, I need to clarify what I mean by biological sex differences. Generally speaking, a person's sex is determined by chromosomes. In humans, each cell normally contains 23 pairs of chromosomes. Twenty-two of these pairs are the same in males and females; the twenty-third pair contains the sex chromosomes and they are different in males and females. Most people are classified at birth as either female (with two X sex chromosomes and female genitalia) or male (with X and Y sex chromosomes and male genitalia). When people are born with a combination of male and female biological traits, they are considered intersex. Whatever one's sex, chromosomes influence the production of sex hormones and have an impact on physiology—how cells, organs and body systems develop and function.

It is also important that I take this opportunity to explain how the term *biological sex* differs from *gender*. Biological sex and gender are not mutually exclusive, and both influence health. However, sex is considered a biological component, while gender is a social construct that involves cultural, environmental and societal expectations and assumptions.

*Gender identity,* on the other hand, refers to how individual people relate to society's understanding of gender, how they feel inside and how they want to express their gender through personal appearance and behavior.

According to OUTRIGHT International, a nongovernmental organization (NGO) dedicated to LGBTIQ human rights, common gender identities include agender, cisgender, demigender, gender questioning, gender fluid, genderqueer, intergender, multigender, nonbinary, pangender, transgender/trans, gender neutral, femme, butch/masc and boi/boy/tomboy.[1]

Throughout this book, I use the term "women" to include both chromosomal females and transgender women who are not chromosomally female but identify as women. You will see that the research literature and other sources frequently use gender and sex as synonyms when they shouldn't. All I can do is try to keep the distinctions clear.

Biological sex, gender and gender identity, as well as race and other demographic characteristics, all play roles in women's health. There are large data gaps in knowledge about everything from the right medication dosages for women's bodies to how symptoms manifest in men and women.

For transgender women, there is also a widespread lack of knowledge[2] among doctors about how to address medical issues that relate to gender-affirming care and other health issues that are impacted by medical transition.[3] In addition, transgender women are at risk of being refused treatment. Few groups experience such significant barriers to healthcare, and yet their struggles are largely unnoticed. There is another major area where ignorance and bias have prevailed. We still don't have a complete, science-based understanding of the effects of racial and ethnic inequity on health outcomes and how racial and ethnic inequity interacts with biological sex differences. What we do know is that inequity—social, economic and educational—impacts health. We also know that in some instances race impacts health biologically. These disparities need to be explored and understood so that everyone can receive appropriate care.

In the 1980s, when the Society for Women's Health Research (SWHR) was powering up, women were struggling mightily to attain equal status in all aspects of American society. Some critics of our work said our emphasis on sex differences research could be used to justify discrimination. My response was (and remains): How can the repression of research possibly be a better course of action? We have no choice but to do the work, be honest about the outcomes and make treatment and health policy decisions based on those realities.

Women need to be treated equitably not only in their professional and personal lives but also in their interactions with healthcare providers and in the work done by medical researchers. Without health equity, women cannot receive the same health benefits as men.

It has been challenging to get researchers and practitioners, research and medical institutions and medication and device manufacturers to accept this. The journey toward sex and gender health equity in prevention, diagnosis and treatment is still ongoing. This book is the story of why it was—and still is—so important to do research specific to women.

When you are done reading this book, it is my hope that you will feel empowered to ask these questions of healthcare providers, whether you are a woman patient or a man helping a woman partner, friend or family member:

- Are you aware of all the research being done on sex differences?
- Was this device tested on women?
- Was this medication tested on women for appropriate dosage, side effects and risk factors?

We need to insist that government agencies, pharmaceutical companies, research universities and medical schools expand their commitment to sex-based health research and care. But as important, we need to take our fight to improve the quality of care for women directly to healthcare practitioners.

To help you accomplish this goal—and to keep the fire lit under the medical community's feet—I am delighted to introduce you to many of the women and men in medicine, social policy, government and the pharmaceutical industry who are working to convince the medical and research establishment that there are sex differences and they must be acknowledged and explored.

## CHAPTER 1

# The History of the Mystery

## Medical Discrimination Against Females Through the Ages

If society will not admit of woman's free development, then
society must be remodeled.

> —*Elizabeth Blackwell, the first woman to
> become a medical doctor in the United States*

The female body has been viewed with awe and fear for millennia. Twenty-three hundred years ago, the philosopher Aristotle wrote that female genitalia is "turn'd outside in."[1] While the Greeks appreciated that this bewildering inversion allowed for the miracle of childbirth, it did nothing to stop them from asserting the indisputable superiority of the male and his sperm.

Five hundred years later, the Greek physician Galen (129–216 AD) constructed his understanding of female biochemistry, anatomy and health on the foundation laid by Hippocrates (the fourth century BC Greek physician), Plato (Aristotle's teacher) and Aristotle. In his work *On the Usefulness of the Parts of the Body,* Galen used the ancient Greek notions of the four basic qualities of the body—hot, cold, wet and dry—to affirm Aristotle's contention that females are less perfect than males. He attributed females' deficiencies to the fact that females are colder of nature than males because their "parts" are within, unlike males', which are properly outside. Galen's analysis of women's bodily deficiencies and inferiority permeated Western concepts of sexual identity and medicine right up to the Industrial Revolution—and beyond.

For millennia, hysteria—the Greek term for "uterus"—was seen as the proper diagnosis for almost every female complaint, from chronic pain to digestive woes, palpitations, fainting, headaches and aching joints. The powers that be believed strenuous activity—physical or mental—would inflame the ovaries and uterus and imperil a female's delicate constitution. Having a uterus defined females' function, and any disease or illness a female had was thought to be caused by their (glorious but dirty) reproductive mysteries and powers.

As the authors of *Women and Hysteria in the History of Mental Health* put it so aptly: "Hysteria is undoubtedly the first mental disorder attributable to women, accurately described in the second millennium BC, and until Freud considered an exclusively female disease. Over 4,000 years of history, this disease . . . was cured with herbs, sex or sexual abstinence, punished and purified with fire for its association with sorcery. . . . [E]ven at the end of the 19th century, scientific innovation had still not reached some places, where the only known therapies were those proposed by Galen."[2]

Speaking of the end of the nineteenth century, in the United States on March 3, 1873, Congress passed the Comstock Act, which stated that contraceptives were obscene and illicit. It became a federal offense to send birth control through the mail or across state lines. As late as the 1960s, 30 states had laws on their books that obstructed the sale and advertisement of birth control to one degree or another. And unfortunately this inclination to repress the use of contraception—and block reproductive healthcare for women—is still going on today.

Then during the twentieth century, several studies suggested there was a decline in diagnoses of hysteria in Western countries and an increase in diagnoses in non-Western countries.[3] Racism combined with misogyny transferred faulty opinions about females' biological inclination for hysteria from Western (read "white") to non-Western (read "people of color") females.

### RECENT HISTORY: MORE RETRO THAN REVOLUTIONARY

In the late twentieth century many missteps were made before hysteria was dropped as an explanation for women's health problems. One of the most damaging was taken in 1977 when the Food and Drug Administration (FDA) issued *General Considerations for the Clinical*

*Evaluation of Drugs.* It banned females with "childbearing potential" from participating in phases 1 and 2 of drug trials, which evaluate toxicity and safe dosages, in order to protect fetuses and reduce liability.[4] The guideline warned that fetuses could unintentionally be exposed to a drug if their mothers did not know they were pregnant when they participated in a drug trial. In practice, researchers and industry professionals assumed that all females should be excluded from all clinical trials.[5] And they were, for years.

As Sherry Marts, PhD, who was vice president for scientific affairs at SWHR for 10 years and acted as the executive director of the Organization for the Study of Sex Differences, sums it up: "You could have been a lesbian nun and they wouldn't have let you into a clinical trial."

This prohibition came in the wake of two drugs and a device that had serious negative side effects for women and their children. The drugs and device were used by women but had never been reliably tested on them. You would hope the rule makers at the FDA would have looked at these horrible outcomes and thought, "We should do more testing on female cells, female lab animals and, in some circumstances, on women." They didn't. Instead, the acknowledged risks to women and their children caused just the opposite response.

The drugs that harmed women and their offspring were diethylstilbestrol (DES) and thalidomide, and the device was the Dalkon Shield.

### ABOUT DES

DES is a synthetic form of estrogen.[6] In 1941, the FDA approved DES for use by females to manage menopause symptoms, suppress breast milk after birth and treat chronic vaginal dryness.

In the late 1940s, Harvard conducted trials of DES in pregnant females. Despite the fact that the studies were conducted without control groups, the researchers concluded that DES was effective for a variety of pregnancy complications and resulted in a "healthier maternal environment."[7] In 1947, the FDA approved marketing DES to prevent miscarriages. That approval remained in effect until 1971, when additional studies linked DES to an increase in females' risk for breast cancer and problems during pregnancy such as miscarriage and preeclampsia. In addition, DES put women's female children at risk for reproductive problems, breast cancer and a rare cancer that affects the kidneys and reproductive organs. Male children were at risk for epididymal cysts on the testicles.[8] When the risks of DES to women and their children became clear, the FDA issued a drug bulletin saying that DES is contraindicated for use during pregnancy.

Also in 1971, a study reported that DES was an effective postcoital contraceptive, spurring the off-label use of DES as an emergency contraceptive pill on many college campuses. In 1975, in part to stop its off-label use, the FDA approved DES as a contraceptive in emergency situations, such as rape and incest. However, the FDA reversed its position and withdrew approval later that year.

By the late 1970s, DES was only approved to treat postmenopausal breast cancer and metastatic prostate cancer and for postpartum lactation suppression. In 1978, the FDA banned the use of DES for postpartum lactation suppression. Finally, in 1985, the FDA listed DES as a known carcinogen, though FDA approval was not withdrawn until September 2000.[9]

## ABOUT THALIDOMIDE

Thalidomide was first marketed—no prescription needed—in the late 1950s by the West German company Chemie Grünenthal as a flu remedy, sedative, tranquilizer and sleeping pill. The idea of using it to ease morning sickness came later. In April 1958, Distillers Company started marketing thalidomide in the United Kingdom. Eventually the drug was sold around the globe under about 40 different names.

The drug was never approved in the United States, but up to 20,000 Americans were given thalidomide in the 1950s and 1960s as part of two clinical trials operated by the pharmaceutical companies Richardson-Merrell and Smith, Kline & French. The US Thalidomide Survivors organization says an estimated 2.5 million doses of thalidomide were supplied to more than 1,200 doctors in the United States under the guise of conducting a clinical trial that was, in reality, a marketing campaign.[10]

Thalidomide never obtained FDA approval, thanks to an FDA employee named Frances Oldham Kelsey, PhD, who repeatedly asked the company for thalidomide lab studies on pregnant animals. The company never complied and never received the go-ahead from her. (Dr. Kelsey received the President's Award for Distinguished Federal Civilian Service from John F. Kennedy in 1962.)

Nonetheless, the manufacturer told physicians that the medication presented no risk to pregnant women or their fetuses. In truth, when taken between the fourth and eighth week of gestation, thalidomide caused fetal and infant deaths, and many babies who survived were born with malformed or missing limbs and damage that affected various organ systems, such as ears, eyes and brain, as they grew up.

Today, thalidomide is approved only for the treatment of leprosy and plasma cell myeloma, with a boxed warning that the drug is contraindicated in pregnant people.[11]

### ABOUT THE DALKON SHIELD

In 1971, an intrauterine device (IUD) called the Dalkon Shield came on the market.[12] The device was not subject to FDA approval because medical devices were not regulated by the FDA at that time. The sales pitch was that it was safer than the newly developed oral contraceptives. In the first three years it was available, the Dalkon Shield was implanted in more than 2.2 million females.

Pretty quickly, the Dalkon Shield was linked to pelvic inflammatory disease, or infection of the uterus, fallopian tubes, ovaries or pelvis. In addition, because the device sometimes failed to block conception, some women became pregnant while using it. The Dalkon Shield also increased their risk of developing sepsis and infections of the fetus and placenta.

In 1974, *Obstetrics and Gynecology* published several studies on the increased risk of septic pregnancies associated with the Dalkon Shield. A year later, the Centers for Disease Control and Prevention published a study stating that the Dalkon Shield came with a higher risk of a woman dying from her pregnancy or spontaneously aborting her fetus than was associated with other IUDs.[13]

After the publication of those studies, A. H. Robins Company discontinued production of the Dalkon Shield, and in 1976, Congress amended the Food, Drug, and Cosmetic Act, adding medical device amendments that required testing and approval of medical devices, including IUDs.[14]

But it was not until October 1984 that the company advised those still using the Dalkon Shield to have it removed. In 1985, after 9,500 cases had been settled or taken to court, the company filed for bankruptcy and $2.3 billion was made available to settle thousands of pending cases.[15]

## EVOLVING: HYSTERIA IS DROPPED AS A LEGITIMATE DIAGNOSIS

It's hard to believe it wasn't until 1980 that hysterical neurosis—the catchall for every female ailment—was finally deleted from the

*Diagnostic and Statistical Manual of Mental Disorders, Third Edition* (*DSM-III*)—the American Psychiatric Association's (APA) bible for the diagnosis of psychiatric disorders.

Following that flash of enlightenment, the next decade saw remarkable efforts by female physicians, lawmakers and activists to wake up the medical and research establishment to the folly of assuming female's biological differences were confined to reproduction.

That journey paralleled mine. While I was in graduate school studying to get my master of social work, I interned at the APA. I was eventually hired as assistant director of government relations, a lobbyist for mental health issues in both the House and Senate.

While at the APA, I became friendly with a number of female psychiatrists and learned about the difficulties they faced in acquiring tenure and getting published in journals. I also started to hear about the lack of females in clinical trials. These mental health professionals specifically talked about depression and how it affected females two to three times more often than males—and yet females were not included in research.

This was my first introduction to sex discrimination in medicine. I began to see that, in addition to discrimination in researching and treating mental illnesses, issues such as abortion, contraception and nonreproductive illnesses in females were being ignored. I was privileged to witness various bureaucracies begin to acknowledge that change was essential.

## THE SOCIETY FOR THE ADVANCEMENT OF WOMEN'S HEALTH RESEARCH ENTERS THE FRAY

In 1985, Florence Haseltine, MD, PhD, was appointed director of the Center for Population Research at the National Institute of Child

Health and Human Development (NICHD). Her role was to champion the field of obstetrics and gynecology. "When I got to there [NIH], OB/GYN just was not considered a real field," she has said.[16] There was little to no focus on conditions other than pregnancy that affected females, such as fibroids, endometriosis and ovarian cancer.

While she was working at NICHD, Dr. Haseltine commuted between Washington, DC, and New Haven, Connecticut, where her family lived. Congresswoman Rosa DeLauro (D-CT), who represented that district, was making the same commute. The two became friends.

Representative DeLauro was diagnosed with ovarian cancer in 1986. Over the next several years, Dr. Haseltine took it upon herself to work with Rosa to find the most effective treatment. She discovered a shocking lack of information and felt that something had to be done. So, in 1989, she organized a meeting on women's health at the American College of Obstetricians and Gynecologists.

As Dr. Haseltine recalled in *The Renaissance Woman in Medicine Oral History Project*, "The first meeting . . . was held in the boardroom of the American College of OB-GYN around their uterus-shaped table. I kid you not. I've been told that doesn't exist anymore, but that's too bad, because it was a nice-looking table. But it was funny . . . [because of] where it was."[17]

Representatives from a wide range of specialties, including osteoporosis, dermatology and cardiology, were brought together to talk to each other about women's health. I was pleased to participate in the event.

It was an eye-opening experience, as the attendees shared their insights—or lack of insights—into the health of women. The subject of sex and gender differences in medicine beyond reproductive issues had never been so publicly discussed before. One of the most fascinating remarks came from a dermatologist who said that trials of skin-related products were all conducted on men.

That meeting laid the groundwork for the formation of the Society for the Advancement of Women's Health Research (SAWHR). Because of my work with the APA and on Capitol Hill, I was invited to be on the new (and revolutionary) organization's board.

Around the same time, Dr. Haseltine decided she needed to address the lack of information about women's health within NICHD. She contacted a PR company, Bass & Howes, to seek advice on how to encourage research on conditions that affect females unrelated to pregnancy and reproduction. Their advice was to not concentrate solely on NICHD, but on all of the National Institutes of Health (NIH).

To promote that broad initiative, members of SAWHR's board scheduled a meeting with the executive director of the Congressional Caucus for Women's Issues. We discussed meeting with representatives who had jurisdiction over the NIH and requesting that the Government Accounting Office (GAO) investigate whether females were being included in all research conducted by the NIH.

While we were meeting, members of the Caucus for Women's Issues discovered there had been a 1985 Public Health Service Task Force on Women's Health Issues report, and that it had noted the lack of research on females' health. It also stated that women were being shortchanged on the quality of health information and care they received.

That such an engaged group of women didn't know the report even existed reveals how little attention was paid to early efforts to address sex differences in healthcare and how difficult it would be going forward to get women's health issues the recognition they deserved.

The much-ignored report recommended that biomedical and behavioral research should be expanded to ensure a "focus on conditions and diseases unique to or more prevalent in females of all ages." That included contraception for females and males, breast cancer, lupus and other arthritic conditions, osteoporosis and certain mental health disorders. The report also highlighted the need for research that clarified how behavioral and social factors interact with biological factors to affect the health of females over their lifetimes.

This led the SAWHR, the Congressional Caucus for Women's Issues and Congressman Henry Waxman (D-CA) to request a report from the GAO on whether the NIH was following the task force's recommendations and encouraging the inclusion of females in clinical research. The resulting GAO report revealed that the NIH had made little progress.

## THE SOCIETY FOR THE ADVANCEMENT OF WOMEN'S HEALTH RESEARCH BECOMES THE SOCIETY FOR WOMEN'S HEALTH RESEARCH

In 1990, I suggested to the board that Dr. Haseltine transform the volunteer-based SAWHR into the Society for Women's Health Research (SWRH), a powerful lobby for women's health research.

I brought my lobbying skills to the fledgling organization to complement the scientific knowledge of other board members. Because I had directed the APA's political action committee and encouraged the APA to support female candidates, I knew Congresswoman Nancy Pelosi (D-CA), Congresswoman DeLauro and others in government. I also had contacts within the pharmaceutical industry through the APA and with people in the media because of my journalist husband's circle. SWHR quickly became the most aggressive and effective organization advocating for women to be included in all aspects of medical research.

## IT'S NOT ALL IN YOUR HEAD—OR YOUR UTERUS

Dr. Haseltine's unwavering commitment to women's health was enormously influential on the establishment of the NIH's Office of Research on Women's Health (ORWH).[18] Vivian W. Pinn, MD, was the first full-time director of ORWH, starting in 1991, and associate director for Women's Health Research at the NIH, beginning in 1994, until her retirement in 2011.

ORWH had a seven-part mandate.[19] It was designed to (1) "advise the NIH director and staff on matters relating to research on women's health"; (2) "strengthen and enhance research related to diseases, disorders and conditions that affect women"; (3) "ensure that research conducted and supported by NIH adequately addresses issues regarding women's health"; (4) "ensure that women are appropriately represented in biomedical and bio-behavioral research studies supported by the NIH"; (5) "develop opportunities and support for recruitment, retention, reentry and advancement of women in biomedical careers"; (6) "support and advance rigorous research that is relevant to the health of women"; and (7) "ensure NIH-funded research accounts for sex as a biological variable (SABV)."

However, it's important to realize that while inclusion of females in clinical research became NIH policy with the establishment of ORWH in 1990, it was not yet law.

That same year, Bernadine Healy, MD, became the first female NIH director and launched the NIH Women's Health Initiative, a set of clinical trials and an observational study sponsored by the National Heart, Lung, and Blood Institute that focused on exploring ways to help prevent postmenopausal women from developing heart disease, breast and colorectal cancer and osteoporosis.[20] The trials enrolled more than 150,000 postmenopausal women over a period of 15 years. (Disputes over the findings about hormone replacement therapy, or HRT, emerged later and cast a shadow over the whole effort.)

At SWHR, we saw opportunities for increasing research into the health of women—if we could build on the first steps being taken within government organizations.

## ENGAGING THE MEDICAL-INDUSTRIAL COMPLEX

While the federal government was slowly making progress, SWHR created the Corporate Advisory Council to bring together representatives from the pharmaceutical industry—and eventually many biotechnology and medical device companies—to discuss sex differences and what they mean for research, drug and device development and women's health. Several companies set up women's health departments or institutes to focus on these issues and support SWHR's mission. SWHR would not have succeeded without them.

"It was not until the 1990s that there was a real push to involve women in medicine development," says Steve Ubl, president and CEO of Pharmaceutical Research and Manufacturers of America (PhRMA). "Much of this was due to groundwork laid by Phyllis and other early leaders in the field. The spark that started this movement continues to this day. You can see it in our industry as we continue to work to not just increase the enrollment of women in clinical trials but enhance racial and ethnic diversity as well."

Around the same time, SWHR formed a medical health advisory board. We brought in experts from every medical specialty to identify areas in their fields where women's health and biological sex needed to be considered. This segued perfectly into SWHR's first Scientific Advisory Meeting (SAM), Towards a Women's Health Research Agenda, in 1991. That roundtable brought together representatives from 25 medical specialties and professional organizations and SWHR's Corporate Advisory Council. The attendees included 5 foundations, 6 medical societies and 15 corporations, including Ortho Pharmaceutical Corporation, Syntex Laboratories, Inc., and Wyeth-Ayerst.

Also in 1991, the Department of Health and Human Services' newly formed Office on Women's Health (OWH) published the *Action Plan for Women's Health,* which highlighted a wide swath of women's health needs that were being neglected or flat-out dismissed.[21] The action plan set out a two-year goal to increase awareness of women's unique health needs, concerning everything from cervical and breast cancer to osteoporosis, urinary incontinence, heart disease, HIV and depression, as well as the adverse effects of smoking, drinking alcohol and drug abuse on females.

A follow-up report from the GAO found that females were a relatively small proportion of study participants in early toxicity and safety studies.[22] The report echoed earlier findings that drug manufacturers and FDA reviewers did not take full advantage of the data generated in drug trials to learn about the effects of drugs in females and to explore sex difference in dosing. The report even suggested that the FDA was not up to the task of monitoring how many females were enrolled in clinical trials.[23]

Another important leap forward was the launch of the *Journal of Women's Health* in January 1992 by Dr. Haseltine, former SWHR board member Dr. Anne Colston Wentz and publisher Mary Ann Liebert. I joined the board of the journal and was pleased that the first issue featured an introduction about SWHR and a short commentary on women's health issues by then–NIH director Dr. Bernadine Healy.

"Florence introduced me to the Society and their message that women's health is more than OB-GYN," recalls Liebert. "Women's health is its own field. It has to do with women's whole body. It was important that it have its own journal."

We were moving forward aggressively. Over the next decade, SWHR held additional roundtables that focused on the need for more women in academic medicine and health science careers, and SWHR produced a series of recommendations to increase the number of women in these fields. And the government was slowly acknowledging the importance of women's health issues with the establishment at the Department of Health and Human Services (HHS) of the Office on Women's Health, the Office of Research on Women's Health at the NIH and the GAO report that highlighted all the shortcomings that persisted in the analysis of sex differences in research data.

But not everything was going smoothly. I encountered numerous barriers; many male doctors in positions of authority didn't accept the whole concept of sex differences. Now, more than three decades later, we are still struggling to get a full accounting of sex differences in many medical conditions and a recognition that more and better-quality research is needed for women-mostly and women-only conditions. In spring 2023, only 10.8% of the NIH's budget was going to fund research on women's health.

## CHAPTER 2

# Calling Their Bluff

## The Society for Women's Health Research Forces the Issue

If they don't give you a seat at the table, bring a folding chair.

—*Shirley Chisholm*

When Bill Clinton was running for president in 1992, I was asked to hold a meet and greet for his wife, Hillary Clinton. I invited all the women I knew. At one point during the gathering I pulled Hillary aside and told her about my work with the Society for Women's Health Research (SWHR) and said that if she was going around the country talking to women, she might want to talk about women's health. Not long after, I received a call from her campaign office saying that she was definitely interested in talking about women's health and asking me to help with speeches and contacts. At that time, I was also working with Tipper Gore's staff on mental health issues, as I was still employed by the American Psychiatric Association (APA).

I am especially proud that in President Clinton's acceptance speech at the Democratic Convention in New York, he said, "I'm ... committed to mak[ing] sure every American gets the healthcare that saved my mother's life and that women's healthcare gets the same attention as men's." Hillary came over to me at the reception and told me that commitment was because of my input.

At SWHR's next board meeting, I suggested that since the Clintons had made women's health a national issue, we should hire staff, raise funds and become a full-fledged organization dedicated to furthering education, advocacy and research on all conditions that affect women. The rest of the board agreed. So, during this challenging time for women's health initiatives, the Society embarked on a search for someone to head the organization.

Around the same time, I began to think that since I had been in-volved in the Clinton campaign and had been at the APA for a number of years, maybe I would go into the new administration. Republican and Democrat friends who had worked in administrations advised me against it. They didn't think I could tolerate the political bureaucracy. I had to agree.

That made me realize that heading an organization devoted to changing the way health research on women was conducted was a challenge I couldn't pass up. I was fortunate to be selected as the first executive director and then, later, president and CEO of SWHR.

In 1993, I gave my notice to the APA. A few days later, I said to my husband, "I have good news and bad news. The good news is, I was selected as president of the Society, and the bad news is, there isn't any money."

I had no office, no staff, nothing. But I did have contacts at a number of pharmaceutical companies from running the APA's political action committee. Interestingly, several women I knew who worked for pharmaceutical companies didn't realize there was an absence of women in clinical trials, but when I brought it to their attention, they helped get funding from their companies for the Society.

Say what you will about the pharmaceutical industry, but if it wasn't for them, the Society would have ceased to exist.

When I took over leadership of SWHR, there was reason for hope. In 1993, President Clinton saw to the passage of the Women's Health Equity Act, which had been introduced in 1990 and blocked by then-president George H. W. Bush because of its pro-choice provi-sions.[1] The Act was designed to promote greater equity in the delivery of healthcare to women by promoting expanded research on women's health issues and improved access to healthcare services, including pre-ventive health services. Bush had also blocked the Freedom of Choice

Act, which would have codified a woman's right to an abortion, and threatened to veto any bill that didn't align with his administration's stance on abortion.[2] We were contending with a seesaw of delay and progress that would be repeated over the 27 years that I was with SWHR and that continues today.

Seeking to capitalize on the administration's interest in women's health, SWHR's focus for the next two years was on changing the perspective of the medical research and clinical communities.

The first year I was head of the Society, SWHR was instrumental in getting Congress to pass the NIH Revitalization Act of 1993.[3] The new policy required that not only were women and members of minority groups to be included in biomedical and behavioral research supported by the NIH but also that, going forward, all institutes must:

- ensure that women and minorities and their subpopulations are included in all human subject research
- for phase 3 clinical trials, ensure that women and minorities and their subpopulations must be included such that valid analyses of differences in intervention effect can be accomplished
- not allow cost as an acceptable reason for excluding these groups
- initiate programs and support for outreach efforts to recruit these groups into clinical studies.

It also stated that it was of utmost importance that all therapies, treatments and interventions be evaluated in terms of their impact on women, men and members of minority groups. The act made it clear that only then could solid scientific evidence emerge that would allow for improved healthcare and social policies for all.

However, the act, with the subtitle "Clinical Research Equity Regarding Women and Minorities," also specified the following:

> INAPPLICABILITY OF REQUIREMENT—The requirement
> established in subsection (a) regarding women and members of
> minority groups shall not apply to a project of clinical research if
> the inclusion, as subjects in the project, of women and members of
> minority groups, respectively—
> (1) is inappropriate with respect to the health of the subjects;
> (2) is inappropriate with respect to the purpose of the research; or
> (3) is inappropriate under such other circumstances as the
>     Director of NIH may designate.

"Inapplicability of requirement" indeed! What the right hand gives, the left hand takes away—or at least creates a loophole to avoid. A careful reexamination in 2018 of 107 NIH-funded randomized, controlled trials conducted in the United States in 2015, confirms how those loopholes got exploited—and for how long that exploitation had been going on.[4] The researchers found only 26% of the trials reported at least one outcome by sex or explicitly included sex as a covariate in statistical analysis. And the study concluded that, overall, "NIH policies have not resulted in significant increases in reporting results by sex, race, or ethnicity."

Even so, the 1993 NIH Revitalization Act was progress. Following the passage of the act, the NIH published guidelines stating that the institutes would not fund any grant, cooperative agreement or contract or support any intramural project unless it complied with this policy.

In light of the changes at the NIH, that same year the FDA rescinded its 1977 policy mandating that women with childbearing potential be excluded from participating in phase 1 and 2 clinical trials. David Kessler, MD, JD, FDA commissioner, told the *New York Times* that he would send rules to pharmaceutical companies "saying that women simply must be included and we are lifting the 16-year ban we have had on women in early drug trials."[5] Dr. Kessler's special assistant on women's health, Dr. Ruth Merkatz, PhD, RN, FAAN, made sure it was known that up to 50% of drug safety trials had excluded women—with significant consequences for women's health.[6]

In 1994, the Office of Women's Health was established at the FDA, and Dr. Merkatz was named its first director. She noted that the efforts of SWHR staff had been "extremely important, especially to be able to influence members of Congress about the importance of establishing the Office of Women's Health at the FDA."

Marsha Henderson, former associate commissioner for women's health at the FDA, remembers, "The Society is why there are offices for women's health. There is no doubt about it. And they kept pressure on the agency to make sure we got our money."

There also was more activity on the Hill. Rep. Olympia Snowe (R-Maine) introduced the Women's Health Office Act (WHOA) in an effort to "protect and advance the health of women through policy, science and outreach; and to advocate for the participation of women in clinical trials and for sex, gender and subpopulation analyses."[7] Its goal was to secure women's health offices within a wide range of federal agencies.

It required those offices to establish goals and objectives and coordinate activities within their respective departments or agencies that relate to disease prevention, health promotion, service delivery and research concerning women and monitor and coordinate federal and regional activities regarding the health of women. Incidentally, WHOA didn't pass and was reintroduced in every Congress from

1994 to 2009. That was the year SWHR's signature piece of legislation passed, securing the offices of women's health within the NIH, FDA and many other federal agencies.

Then in 1997, the FDA published "Guideline for the Study and Evaluation of Gender Differences in the Clinical Evaluation of Drugs."[8] It provided new guidance on the FDA's expectations regarding inclusion of women in drug development, the analysis of clinical data by sex and the conducting of additional studies on women where indicated.

The next year, working with the acting director of the FDA's Office of Women's Health, Audrey Sheppard, Henderson and the FDA launched the Take Time to Care program, which provides millions of women with health and safety information so they can take charge of their own well-being. Clearly the OWH was a force to be reckoned with.

Henderson recalls that initially the senior executive staff members at the FDA thought the Office of Women's Health should sunset in one year. "We were imposed on the agency. We were not something they thought was necessary," says Henderson. "They thought the lawyers on the [Office of Women's Health] staff could make the legal changes and then the [Office of Women's Health] could just go away." But it didn't.

"Phase 1 for the [Office of Women's Health] was the drafting of regulations and guidelines and developing messaging, mostly to the public, about why [the office] was necessary and what the state of affairs [was] at the time," says Henderson. "In phase 2, the goal was to try to use the small budget we had for grants. But it wasn't enough money to really receive proposals from the outside, like the NIH could. Nothing was well-defined, and it turned out that if you put the word 'woman' in front of whatever the title of your grant proposal was you could get some money."

### EXPANDING SWHR'S REACH

The success of the first Scientific Advisory Meeting (SAM) in 1991 spurred the Society to extend our reach beyond Washington, DC. A number of the Society's board members were affiliated with or had colleagues at universities, and they helped arrange SAMs at academic institutions around the country.

Each session focused on whatever evidence on sex differences in medical science was available. Most of the data came from unexpected results in research or treatment where sex differences were inadvertently or serendipitously revealed. The Society looked at everything from cardiovascular issues to bone health to sports injuries, cancer, violence against women, depression and substance abuse. This was a major shift, expanding the conversation beyond women's health issues that were related to reproduction.

As Janine Clayton, MD, associate director for research on women's health and director of the Office of Research on Women's Health at the NIH, would put it some time later (but it applies to what was going on then), "We were looking not at women's health but the health of women."

We met with the presidents of many universities and other executives—all of whom were male in those days—to plan the Scientific Advisory Meetings. What struck me was that if the man we met with had a daughter in medical school or who was already practicing medicine, he was much more open to our message. Otherwise, there was a great deal of skepticism, and we had to work to convince them to agree to hold the meetings at their institutions.

These meetings convinced many in the medical research community of the importance of considering sex in research and clinical practice. At the same time, they also revealed the glaring fact that there was still an enormous amount of education needed before researchers across the board would embrace the concept of sex differences and understand the importance of studying them in the lab and in clinical trials.

"I have been involved with the Society and Phyllis almost since the beginning," says Nanette Wenger, MD, who coined the term "bikini medicine" and is a clinical cardiologist and professor emerita at Emory University School of Medicine, consultant at the Emory Heart and Vascular Center and founding consultant at Emory Women's Heart Center. "I chaired the board of SWHR for two terms when the whole concept of sex differences was very new and very few individuals in public service or medicine acknowledged it. Getting people to pay attention to the concept of sex differences was a struggle. The response of the scientific community was very, very delayed."

The Society was intent on tackling the big health issues confronting women. In February 1993, we convened a menopause workshop that looked at the neurological, cardiovascular, social and psychological changes that are associated with menopause, as well as menopause's potential effect on women's risk factors for osteoporosis and endometrial and breast cancer. We published "Women's Health Research and Menopause: A Dialogue Among Public Policy, Community, and Health Leaders" to lay out the scope of what was covered at the meeting.

It's hard to believe now, 30 years later, that we were being daring and audacious to look at women's reproductive biology scientifically, instead of dismissing it as a cause and manifestation of emotional disturbance—but we were bold and proud of it.

In June 1993, we held the third SAM, addressing the effect of the environment on women's health. That was followed a year later by SWHR's fourth SAM, which turned a spotlight on the health needs of women between the ages of 18 and 24. We held focus groups on college campuses and uncovered a lot of misinformation about diet, physical fitness, partner violence, sexual health and drug use that was harming young women. As a result, we decided to team up with the US Public Health Service's Office on Women's Health to create a video program called *Get Real: Straight Talk About Women's Health.*[9] It presented young adult women across the country with facts about eating disorders, nutrition, exercise, alcohol and substance abuse, violence, contraception, sexually transmitted diseases and smoking.

At the same time, the FDA's associate commissioner for women's health, Henderson, started doing extensive community-related outreach. "We talked with any group that had an interest in the health of women—consumer advocacy groups, racial and ethnic groups, insurance companies," she recalls. "Our office developed a strong network of supporters for our mission. However, there were times when our budget was at risk. Whenever this happened, we knew that we had a secret weapon to protect our program. It was Phyllis. She became the most recognizable person in the movement and the only one who could pick up the phone, call the commissioner (no matter the party affiliation), and she/he would answer the call directly."

There was even more federal interest and action: By 1994, the Congressional Caucus for Women's Issues had grown from 15 women to 47. It was led by co-chairs Congresswomen Pat Schroeder (D-CO) and Olympia Snowe (R-ME). They expanded the issues the caucus addressed to include women's health, childcare, family and medical leave and violence against women. It was during this time that Congress passed the Family and Medical Leave Act, the Violence Against Women Act, and childcare legislation and expressed significantly more support for women's health research.

Always looking for our next sortie into the bastions of power, the Society focused on how we can do more to educate the scientific and medical community, as well as healthcare providers and the general public, about the existence and importance of sex differences.

Auspiciously, at the Society's next annual board meeting, Queta Bond, PhD, the Institute of Medicine's executive officer from 1989 to 1994, suggested the Society go to the Institute of Medicine and request a report on women in clinical trials and sex differences. That launched the Society into a partnership with the Institute of Medicine. And it heralded my multiple-year battle to enlist government agencies and institutes, along with pharma and healthcare organizations, as supporters of this report.

## CHAPTER 3

# Every Cell Has a Sex

## The Institute of Medicine Joins with the Society for Women's Health Research to Lead the Way

The secret of change is to focus all of your energy not on fighting the old, but on building the new.

—*Socrates*

had heard of the Institute of Medicine (IOM) but really didn't know how they operated or whether they would be interested in sex differences. Nevertheless, I made an appointment with Andrew M. Pope, PhD, director of health science policy at the IOM. The Society wanted to see if the IOM would initiate a study on the importance of sex differences in medicine that would get the attention of federal health bureaucracies as well as the scientific and medical communities.

It turned out there was already some interest in the topic at the IOM. In September 1992, in response to a request from the National Institutes of Health (NIH) Office of Research on Women's Health, the IOM convened the Committee on the Ethical and Legal Issues Relating to the Inclusion of Women in Clinical Studies. The 16 members of the committee had backgrounds in bioethics, law, epidemiology and biostatistics, public health policy, obstetrics and gynecology, clinical research, pharmaceutical development, social and behavioral sciences and clinical evaluative sciences. They published *Women and Health Research: Ethical and Legal Issues of Including Women in Clinical Studies* in 1994 with the goal of increasing researchers' awareness of the importance of including women in medical research.[1]

The National Academies website, where you can download the report for free, says the publication "documents the historical shift from a paternalistic approach by researchers toward women and a disproportionate reliance on certain groups for research to one that emphasizes proper access for women as subjects in clinical studies in order to ensure that women receive the benefits of research."[2]

The publication addressed challenges to equity in four areas:

**Scientific**—Do practical aspects of scientific research work at cross-purposes to gender equity? Focusing on drug trials, the authors identified rationales for excluding people from research based on demographics.

**Social and Ethical**—The authors offered compelling discussions of subjectivity in science, the evidence for male bias, and issues related to race and ethnicity, as well as the recruitment, retention and protection of research participants.

**Legal**—*Women and Health Research* reviewed federal research policies that affect the inclusion of women and examined the basis for researchers' fears about liability, citing court cases.

**Risk**—The authors focused on risk to reproduction and offspring in clinical drug trials, exploring how risks can be identified for study participants, who should make the assessment of risk and benefit for participation in a clinical study and how potential legal issues might be addressed.

Nonetheless, the concept of sex differences wasn't part of the daily thought processes at the IOM. When I met with Dr. Pope, he was polite but a bit wary.

"Phyllis approached me with this new idea, and I didn't know what to make of her," Dr. Pope says, looking back on our first meeting in 1994. "I was nervous about advocating for research that was proposed by an advocacy group like SWHR. Our work is supposed to be for the federal government, and it can't happen without support from other government organizations. But the concept of sex as a determinant of health was an interesting idea. I don't know that I was totally sold on the whole idea, but it was new, so I went for it. I said I would talk to the NIH."

He agreed to work with us and it was the start of a long and winding road that we—and our two organizations—happily traveled together. The immediate challenge was finding government and private sponsors who would fund the research. Dr. Pope explained that as a federal agency, the IOM could only consider requests from other government entities, not a nonprofit organization like the Society. Additionally, it would cost $350,000 to get the research going. That was more money than the annual budget for the Society for Women's Health Research (SWHR).

I had to raise, or help raise, the funding. Some supplemental funds could come from private sources, but the majority of the money had to come from government entities. While Dr. Pope started to try to find support from the Food and Drug Administration (FDA), Centers for Disease Control and Prevention (CDC), Department of Health and Human Services (HHS) and the Office of Research on Women's Health (ORWH), SWHR looked for potential corporate sponsors.

I spoke with SWHR's major funders, and Johnson & Johnson and Unilever both agreed to supply the full amount allowed from private funding.

Then Dr. Pope and I went to medical and scientific governmental entities to request funding for this commission. I knocked on the door of most of the 27 NIH institutes. That effort was mostly unsuccessful.

Part of the problem, I was told later, was that the head of ORWH called NIH directors and told them not to contribute to the study. ORWH also refused to be the government sponsor for the IOM report.

Nonetheless, several institutes ended up endorsing and supporting the IOM effort: the National Institute of Drug Abuse (NIDA), where I knew the staff from my years at the American Psychiatric Association, and the National Institute of Mental Health and the National

Institute of Environmental Health (NIEH), because I knew their directors personally and was on NIEH's patient advocacy commission.

Finally, we had funding from three NIH institutes, Johnson & Johnson and Unilever, but we were still short.

## EVEN THE RATS WERE MALE

Dr. Pope contacted some science and research agencies and asked if they would provide funds too. As it turned out, they understood that the science of sex differences was a critical part of their mission to conduct quality research. They told Dr. Pope they were in—but only if the commission explored sex differences in basic science that was conducted in the lab using animals and cells. This turned out to be the best thing that could have happened.

SWHR continued to focus on the inclusion of women and minorities in clinical trials and the IOM commission expanded their focus to include the importance of sex differences in lab-based research. Without that we wouldn't have *Sex Cells!*

However, there was still one more step. While we had sufficient funding, we still needed a government entity to sponsor the commission. I asked Wanda Jones, DrPH, MD, director of women's health at HHS, and she agreed.

Finally, we had the funding and a government sponsor.

Ultimately support for the project came from SWHR, and according to the National Library of Medicine,[3] the US Department of Health and Human Services (Office on Women's Health, National Institutes of Health Office of Research on Women's Health, National Institute of Environmental Health Sciences, National Institute on Drug Abuse, National Institute of Mental Health, US Food and Drug

Administration, Centers for Disease Control and Prevention), the National Science Foundation, the Environmental Protection Agency, the National Aeronautics and Space Administration, the Research Foundation for Health and Environmental Effects, Ortho-McNeil/Johnson & Johnson and the Unilever United States Foundation. In addition, the project was "approved by the governing board of the National Research Council, whose members are drawn from the councils of the National Academy of Sciences, the National Academy of Engineering, and the Institute of Medicine."

In 1995, the IOM, with SWHR as a partner, submitted the final proposal to Congress to get the go-ahead.

It would be almost seven years after I first met with Dr. Pope that the report would finally come out.

## THE INSTITUTE OF MEDICINE REPORT IS RELEASED

In 2001, the IOM published the ground-shaking report *Exploring the Biological Contributions to Human Health: Does Sex Matter?*[4] The IOM was supposed to hold a press conference announcing the release, and we had obtained funds from Johnson & Johnson to print up bound copies of the report's executive summary to distribute to the press, agencies, anyone interested—but for some reason (I still don't know why), the IOM canceled their press briefing. So the Society held one. The journalist Susan Dentzer interviewed me and helped spread the word.

## THE REPORT'S CONCLUSIONS

Mary-Lou Pardue, PhD, Boris Magasanik professor at the Massachusetts Institute of Technology, chaired the IOM panel that wrote the report. In the 2001 fall/winter issue of the National Academies' *In Focus* magazine she said, "It is widely known that studies on variables such as sex, age, race, or ethnicity have all too often been biased and have led to discriminatory practices."[5] And she laid out the basic findings of the IOM report:

- It would benefit women and men if biomedical researchers started paying more attention to sex differences.
- Doing so could identify new ways to improve the way diseases are diagnosed and treated.
- Sex differences should be studied on a cellular level to determine the influence of sex on how bodily systems function and susceptibility to disease.
- Until being male or female is routinely considered when designing studies and sex differences are routinely reported, medical care will miss many chances to improve women's and men's health.

Now, decades later, the quest has expanded from focusing on science-based, sex-specific research to advocating that both research and clinical practice be driven by awareness of the importance of sex differences.

"These days," says Dr. Pope, "it's hard to look back and recall what the mental framework was at the time. Now we understand that there was a bias in medical research and female animals were excluded from basic science because they were thought to be hysterical because of their cycles! Ha! The bias permeated clinical trials *and* lab studies."

## THE IOM STUDY DETAILS

On the basis of its review, the committee identified research gaps and developed recommendations to facilitate scientific investigations of sex differences. Their 14 recommendations distill the important facets of the report.[6]

Recommendation 1: Promote research on sex at the cellular level. The committee recommends that research be conducted to

- determine the functions and effects of X-chromosome- and Y-chromosome-linked genes in somatic cells as well as germ-line cells,
- determine how genetic sex differences influence other levels of biological organization (cell, organ, organ system, organism), including susceptibility to disease, and
- develop systems that can identify and distinguish between the effects of genes and the effects of hormones.

Recommendation 2: Study sex differences from womb to tomb. The committee recommends that researchers and those who fund research focus on the following areas:

- inclusion of sex as a variable in basic research designs,
- expansion of studies to reveal the mechanisms of intrauterine effects, and
- encouragement of studies at different stages of the life span to determine how sex differences influence health, illness and longevity.

Recommendation 3: Mine cross-species information.

- Researchers should choose models that mirror human sex differences and that are appropriate for the human conditions being addressed. Given the interspecies variation, the mechanisms of sex differences in nonhuman primates may be the best mimics for some mechanisms of sex differences in humans. Continued development of appropriate animal models, including those involving nonhuman primates, should be encouraged and supported under existing regulations and guidelines.

- Researchers should be alert to unexpected phenotypic sex differences resulting from the production of genetically modified animals.

Recommendation 4: Investigate natural variations.

- Examine genetic variability, disorders of sex differentiation, reproductive status, and environmental influences to better understand human health.
- Naturally occurring variations provide useful models that can be used to study the influences and origins of a range of factors that influence sex differences.

Recommendation 5: Expand research on sex differences in brain organization and function.

New technologies make it possible to study sex-differential environmental and behavioral influences on brain organization and function and to recognize modulators of brain organization and function. Explore innovative ways to expand the availability of and reduce the cost of new technologies.

Recommendation 6: Monitor sex differences and similarities for all human diseases that affect both sexes. Investigators should

- consider sex as a biological variable in all biomedical and health related research; and
- design studies that will control for exposure, susceptibility, metabolism, physiology (cycles), and immune response variables; consider how ethical concerns (e.g., risk of fetal injury) constrain study designs and affect outcomes; and detect sex differences across the life span.

Recommendation 7: Clarify use of the terms *sex* and *gender*. Researchers should specify in publications their use of the terms *sex* and *gender*. To clarify usage and bring some consistency to the literature, the committee recommends the following:

- In the study of human subjects, the term *sex* should be used as a classification, generally as male or female, according to the reproductive organs and functions that derive from the chromosomal complement.
- In the study of human subjects, the term *gender* should be used to refer to a person's self-representation as male or female, or how that person is responded to by social institutions on the basis of the individual's gender presentation.
- In most studies of nonhuman animals the term *sex* should be used.

Recommendation 8: Support and conduct additional research on sex differences.

Recommendation 9: Make sex-specific data more readily available.

Recommendation 10: Determine and disclose the sex of origin of biological research materials.

Recommendation 11: Longitudinal studies should be conducted and should be constructed so that their results can be analyzed by sex.

Recommendation 12: Identify the endocrine status of research subjects (an important variable that should be considered, when possible, in analyses).

Recommendation 13: Encourage and support interdisciplinary research on sex differences.

Recommendation 14: Reduce the potential for discrimination based on identified sex differences.

Without the IOM's report, the expansion of medical research and clinical practice to include sex differences in female cells, animals and humans might never have happened or certainly would have taken many more years. This report launched the discussion of sex differences that continues today.

## CHAPTER 4

# Evolution of the Revolution

## From Scientific Advisory Meetings to the Founding of the Organization for the Study of Sex Differences

Science gathers knowledge faster than society gathers wisdom.

—*Isaac Asimov*

During the almost seven years it took for the IOM report to be funded, written and published, the Society for Women's Health Research (SWHR) was dedicated to increasing scientific knowledge about sex differences.

In 1995, the Society hosted its fifth annual Scientific Advisory Meeting (SAM), "Gender-Based Biology: What Does It Mean and Why Does It Matter?" The meeting looked at sex differences in neurobiology, language ability after stroke, autoimmunity and osteoporosis. After the meeting, SWHR published several articles about sex differences in the August issue of the *Journal of Women's Health,* the Society's official journal.

Thirty years ago, even the Society used *sex* and *gender* interchangeably. That changed, of course, but the melding together of those two concepts and the erasure of people with nonbinary gender identities is something we must acknowledge and apologize for.

That was also the year Roberta Biegel, MA, who had worked as the legislative aide for the co-chair's liaison with the Congressional Caucus for Women's Issues, joined the Society as director of government relations, a post she would hold for eight years.

"Until we were aligned with the IOM, no one really took us seriously enough on the issue of sex differences," says Biegel. "But when the Society started working with them and interacting with the FDA, Congress and the NIH, folks paid more attention."

The next year, we held the sixth SAM, on the role of sex-based research in human genetics. We felt that if we could increase the medical and research community's understanding of differences in genetics and inheritance between males and females, that would lay a solid foundation for exploring sex differences in diagnosis, prevention and treatment for a wide range of diseases and conditions for women—and for men.

SWHR's seventh SAM, in October 1997, explored healthcare delivery outcomes. This was a chance to look at what health outcomes are the result of biological sex differences and which the result of differences in medical care that males and females receive for the same conditions and diseases.

In 1998, Dr. Sherry Marts came on board as the Society's vice president for scientific affairs. Dr. Marts directed SWHR programs on research on sex differences and on women's health research, including public education campaigns, scientific meetings and conferences, research support programs and information dissemination. We were establishing ourselves as a formidable force with a staff of seasoned, effective professionals who were determined to change how medical research studied sex differences and clinical practice treated women.

## STEPS FORWARD—AND SIDEWAYS

The concept of sex differences was gaining followers, such as Marianne J. Legato, MD, who launched the Partnership for Women's Health at Columbia University in February 1997. However, Dr. Legato had a publication called *Gender & Health,* when she meant *Sex & Health.* That confusion in language was everywhere.

"I remember working on a trial for HIV prevention, and I went to a conference right after SWHR was pushing the FDA to say they would change the guidelines," recalls Dr. Marts. "The FDA was presenting information on having 'both genders in clinical trials.' I walked up to some man with an FDA identification around his neck and said, 'Why are we talking about gender? This is about biological sex—how a drug affects someone's biology if they are male or female. That's not gender, that's sex.' And the FDA representative told me, 'We had to change it to *gender*. We were told we couldn't send the proposed guidelines to the Hill with the word *sex* in them.' That one thing messed up the literature for years because when they said they were talking about gender differences, they actually meant sex differences!'"

In 1999, based on the Society's eighth SAM in 1998, which looked at neurology, psychiatry, immunology and pharmacology, the Society published "The Sexual Revolution in Science: What Gender-Based Research Is Telling Us" in the *Journal of Investigative Medicine*. The Society, with Dr. Marts's leadership, also increased its efforts on Capitol Hill to make lawmakers aware of the issues surrounding sex differences.

To spur that on, in 2000, the Society established a Women's Health Research Coalition, which brought together more than 600 advocates from academic, medical, science and health organizations, as well as health researchers, healthcare providers and policymakers to advocate for SWHR's legislative initiatives during an annual Capitol Hill Day.

We also hosted the first Women's Health Legislative Strategy Conference, which brought together members of the Congressional Caucus on Women's Issues for a series of strategy meetings that were focused on creating a women's health action plan.

The year 2000 also saw the tenth and final SAM. It was on drug addiction and pain. Two journal articles came out of the meeting and were published in 2004 in the *Journal of Women's Health:* "Women and Tobacco Use"[1] and "Women, Men, and Pain."[2]

While all these positive steps forward were taking place, the Government Accountability Office issued a report stating that National Institutes of Health (NIH) research did in fact include women—but the data weren't analyzed by sex.

## FROM SCIENTIFIC ADVISORY MEETINGS TO
## CONFERENCES ON SEX AND GENE EXPRESSION

Fortunately, in 2000, as the last SAM wound down, SWHR received a three-year grant from Aventis Pharmaceuticals that provided enough funding to establish conferences on Sex and Gene Expression (SAGE). The grant allowed us to pay for presentations, travel, food and lodging for all attendees. With all the other medical and scientific meetings there were, we were concerned no one would come if they had to pay—especially when they didn't even know what sex differences were.

The first SAGE conference, in March of that year, looked at how biological sex influences the expression of genetic information in embryos, children and adults. Dr. Florence Haseltine, founder of SWHR, arranged for a third of the attendees to be students and postdoctoral fellows because it is so important to educate up-and-coming healthcare providers and researchers about sex differences. All future SAGE conferences would be planned with the same goal: to get the next generation of people in the medical field in tune with the importance of sex differences in research and clinical care.

In 2003, we increased the Society's depth of expertise. Dr. Marts was joined by Martha Nolan as vice president of public policy at the Society. "Within months of my starting to work at SWHR," recalls Nolan, "as a member of the Ad Hoc Coalition for Medical Research, I participated in meetings with the various NIH institute directors to learn about what they were working on and what new research was coming." It showed her just what we were up against.

"In a meeting with the National Institute of Allergy and Infectious Diseases, I had the opportunity to ask Dr. Anthony Fauci if he had ever looked at whether there were sex differences in the responses to vaccines. His response was an adamant no, and to be honest, I felt like I had my head handed to me, like it wasn't a worthy question. He shut me down.

"I don't tell this story to poke at Dr. Fauci, who is remarkably intelligent, but to put it in the context of the time. Phyllis and all of us at the Society were constantly getting the same kind of response from other scientists. Variations on my question came up over and over and so did the dismissal of the importance of sex differences. But we were determined. We recognized that it takes time to implement such changes, and we were determined to make sure they did get adopted."

It was amazing that even men as smart as Dr. Fauci were resistant to the idea of sex differences. I invited him to the Society's annual dinner every year, and he always had an excuse not to come.

### EXPANDING ACADEMIC INVOLVEMENT

Much important work was made possible by a $1 million grant from Ortho-McNeil. SWHR used it to establish the Interdisciplinary Science Networks (ISN) in January 2002. Initially called ISIS (Interdisciplinary Studies in Sex Differences) after the Egyptian and Greek goddess of healing, we changed the name when it became associated with a terrorist organization.

To get ISN off the ground, we combed the country to find an interdisciplinary group of scientists whose work or specialty would contribute to the discussion. In the beginning, since sex differences were such a new concept, there were not many scientists to choose from. Some researchers who we thought were targeting important and relevant issues said they'd never considered sex differences.

ISN was the first interdisciplinary network of scholars and researchers in the biomedical sciences to promote collaboration among various disciplines on sex differences and women's health. During the gatherings, the groups looked at knowledge gaps in medical science and proposed research that would help fill them. We had network members submit research proposals that were peer reviewed by other network members, and then the researchers who had submitted the proposal could launch research into the sex differences in a given area.

Examples of the networks that were established include the Brain Network, which ran from 2002 to 2007. It aimed to develop collaborations for research on sex differences in nervous system function and to translate the results of this research into new and improved therapies.

The Metabolism Network ran from 2003 to 2009 and advanced the understanding of sex-dependent differences in energy homeostasis and metabolic disorders. SWHR funded three projects investigating sex differences in this topic, and network members published multiple peer-reviewed articles and presented at two meetings on metabolism.

Another area we focused on was Alzheimer's disease (AD). It was the first time anyone looked at sex differences in AD. Research revealed that women are more susceptible to AD and it progresses more quickly in women. All this was a surprise to the scientists.

Roundtables were also held on sex differences in cardiovascular issues, musculoskeletal health, urological health, exercise, breast cancer and sleep.

While all this was going on, I testified at a 2003 NIH conference following the release of the Women's Health Initiative study of 27,347 US women ages 50–79 who enrolled in the Women's Health Initiative Hormone Trials between 1993 and 1998. The study included 16,608 women with an intact uterus and 10,739 without a uterus for a mean follow-up time of 5.2 years. They received either conjugated equine estrogens (CEE) plus medroxyprogesterone acetate, conjugated equine estrogen, or a placebo. The study participants who were given hormones were on them for an average of three years. They were then tracked for an additional eight years to see what health issues appeared.

The researchers found that among every 10,000 women taking hormones there would be 20 more major illnesses or deaths per year. That translated to a 12% increased risk of developing a major illness or dying if a woman were taking estrogen plus progestin compared to women taking placebo pills.[3] However, the absolute numbers of major illnesses and deaths were lower in women between the ages of 50 and 59 (12 more per year for every 10,000 women).

For women who received hormones, the increased risks of cardio-vascular disease, breast cancer and stroke were thought to outweigh the benefits: control of menopausal symptoms and reduction of os-teoporotic fractures and colorectal cancer. Because of these risks, the trial was stopped prematurely.

The tremendously negative information about hormone replacement therapy (HRT) that the media put out in response to that research caused women to stop HRT and doctors to panic about liability con-cerns. The problem was that although this study included only women, the majority of participants were older postmenopausal women and many were smokers and had diabetes and/or obesity. The analysis also made no distinction about the form of the hormones used, how they were administered or how the administration of them was timed in relationship to menopause. I tried to point that out, without much effect. It took decades for new evidence from better-conducted studies to show that HRT is safe and helps prevent certain health conditions if it is taken during perimenopause and in the years right after meno-pause occurs.[4]

At the Society, we couldn't get a lot of traction around the topic either. When we held a roundtable on HRT that year, we brought together those who were critical of the Women's Health Initiative's findings that HRT was risky and those who were not. Although this was of enormous importance to all women and their health as they age, we were unable to raise additional funds to continue exploring the data.

One piece of good news: In 2002, the NIH established Specialized Centers of Research (SCOR) on Sex Differences,[5] which morphed into the Specialized Centers of Research Excellence (SCORE) on Sex Differences program in 2018.[6] The 2002 program was "the first NIH disease-agnostic P50 centers program on sex differences and funded basic, interdisciplinary, and translational research to improve women's health." These days, each SCORE (there are now 11, including at Mayo Clinic) conducts innovative, complex research into the impact of sex differences on health and well-being. The program has paralleled efforts to increase academic involvement in sex-specific research that SWHR was promoting through the Interdisciplinary Science Networks (ISN) and enhanced the opportunity for research to be done and reported accurately.

## FROM THE CONFERENCE ON SEX AND GENE EXPRESSION TO THE ORGANIZATION FOR THE STUDY OF SEX DIFFERENCES

"At the SAGE Conference in 2006, I told everyone that it was likely our last one," recalls Dr. Marts. "Then, something amazing happened. I was approached by a group who told me they wanted to start a new scientific society and have SAGE be their official conference." The Organization for the Study of Sex Differences (OSSD) was established as a Society program from 2006 to 2012 and then became an independent nonprofit.

The founding members included Drs. Haseltine and Marts, as well as 19 scholars and doctors from around the country. Some were members of SWHR's ISN and SWHR staff.

Kathryn Sandberg, PhD, professor of nephrology and hypertension, vice chair for research at the Department of Medicine at Georgetown University Medical Center and director of the Center for the Study of Sex Differences in Health, Aging and Disease, was the first president. OSSD held its first annual meeting in May 2007. It had panels on "The Impact of Sex and Gender on Musculoskeletal Disorders on Earth and in Space" and "Depression, Anxiety and Schizophrenia and Imprinting and Parent-of-Origin Effects," as well as individual panels on sex differences in autoimmunity, obesity and metabolic disease, pain, lung cancer and behavioral disorders.[7] And that was just the beginning of the remarkable gatherings of experts on every topic impacting sex differences in research and clinical care.

"I go to outcomes first," says Dr. Sandberg. "What we needed to do—and still need to do—is get everybody to be part of the pipeline of treatment discovery, from those doing basic science and conducting clinical trials to people who focus on community health and policy."

Dr. Sandberg's point of view shaped OSSD. The goal of the organization was to foster communication and collaboration between scientists and clinicians of diverse backgrounds. That seemed a powerful way to encourage interdisciplinary research proposals on the biology of sex and gender. In addition, OSSD wanted to explore how new knowledge about sex differences could improve women's and men's on-the-ground healthcare experience. OSSD members also wanted to mentor up-and-coming researchers and clinicians to help them develop ways to explore sex differences—and then apply the knowledge to patients.

After Dr. Marts left, SWHR needed someone to spearhead scientific affairs, which were getting ever more complex. Monica Mallampalli, PhD, MSc, came onboard as vice president of scientific affairs from 2010 to June 2017. According to Dr. Mallampalli, "I provided strategic vision and a leadership role towards developing and executing SWHR's scientific initiatives related to women's health and sex-based biology. I managed and implemented scientific programs pertaining to many disease areas in women's health and primarily oversaw activities of SWHR's interdisciplinary research committees."

The 2010 Affordable Care Act (ACA) also played a big role in furthering the government's commitment to sex differences research and policy. The ACA established several offices of women's health, gave those offices new authority and protected them from being eliminated without the direct approval of Congress. Those offices include the NIH's Office of Research on Women's Health; the Department of Health and Human Services' Office on Women's Health; the Substance Abuse and Mental Health Services Administration's position of associate administrator for Women's Services; the FDA's Office of Women's Health; the Centers for Disease Control and Prevention's Office of Women's Health; the Agency for Healthcare Research and Quality's Office of Women's Health, and Gender Research and the Health Resources and Services Administration's Office of Women's Health.[8] Congress has played a key role in establishing and authorizing offices on women's health in the federal government, in addition to financially supporting their work through federal funding.

"These were exciting times," recalls Nolan. "In 2012, we managed to get an amendment attached to a 'must-pass' bill—the FDA Safety and Innovation Act—on the need for analysis and reporting on demographic data with respect to new drug approvals. This provision has resulted in the agency looking at how well demographic subgroups are represented in the drug approval process, making sure the data is analyzed and then having the results made available on a publicly accessible website called Drug Trials Snapshots."[9]

Nonetheless, getting the top brass at the NIH institutes and elsewhere to understand sex differences and their importance in both clinical and research studies was an ongoing effort.

Francis S. Collins, MD, PhD, director of the NIH, like Dr. Fauci, wasn't a fan of SWHR. He also turned down every invitation to attend our annual dinner until I asked him to give the keynote speech. And he wasn't really getting the whole issue about sex differences.

After the FDA laid the groundwork for the Drug Trials Snapshots website, Dr. Collins was rehearsing with his colleagues for his appearance before the committee that approved NIH budgets. In the rehearsal, he answered a question about studying sex differences in basic science by saying it was too complicated and costly to research sex differences on a basic level—meaning in lab studies and cell-based research.

That wasn't the answer his staff wanted him to give, so they called in Janine Clayton, MD, director of ORWH, to help reshape his responses. They wanted to make sure he would be a strong advocate for the importance of women's place in research and clinical studies.

"I was on the committee that had an oversight role, and I played a role in getting Dr. Collins to change his tune and that moved it forward," recalls Representative Rosa DeLauro. "We were talking back and forth. . . . It was a success."

Ultimately, in his testimony Dr. Collins said, "We have now had extensive conversations with all of the institute directors, the scientific community and my Advisory Committee to the Director, which is my most senior advisory group, about this issue."[10]

Shortly after that, Drs. Collins and Clayton wrote a commentary in *Nature* pledging to improve the balance of male and female subjects in preclinical research supported by the NIH.[11] In the strongly worded piece they said:

Today, just over half of NIH-funded clinical-research participants are women. We know much more about the role of sex and gender in medicine, such as that low-dose aspirin has different preventive effects in women and men, and that drugs such as zolpidem, used to treat insomnia, require different dosing in women and men.

There has not been a corresponding revolution in experimental design and analyses in cell and animal research—despite multiple calls to action. Publications often continue to neglect sex-based considerations and analyses in preclinical studies. Reviewers, for the most part, are not attuned to this failure. The over-reliance on male animals and cells in preclinical research obscures key sex differences that could guide clinical studies. And it might be harmful: women experience higher rates of adverse drug reactions than men do.

The upshot was that going forward, the NIH would require all researchers who received grants to balance their use of male and female animals and cells.

Representative DeLauro, who was the senior Democrat on the subcommittee responsible for funding the Department of Health and Human Services, which includes the NIH, released the following statement:

Today's announcement by Dr. Collins is a great step forward and I welcome the announcement that the NIH will begin addressing gender differences in preclinical trials. We know that every cell has a sex, and that diseases present themselves and evolve differently in women, and that women respond to treatments in different ways. We need to align our research efforts with that reality, in all phases of research, from setting priorities to transferring ideas to markets. Going forward, it is critical that the "balance" Dr. Collins refers to does indeed ensure women are treated on an equal playing field with men.

## A WIDER NET

After 27 years at SWHR, I was considering retiring. During that period, a good friend of mine who was on the board of HealthyWomen asked me if I would meet with their CEO, Beth Battaglino, RN-C. HealthyWomen had been a vital communication and education organization. Moving forward, it was interested in getting involved in policy and advocacy and establishing a presence in Washington.

I thought that working with them could be a way to continue to work in women's health but not have all the responsibilities of a CEO. In 2018, I agreed to come onboard as their senior vice president of science and health policy. I encouraged Battaglino to have a fundraising event to establish a DC presence. It was extremely successful, particularly with FDA commissioner Scott Gottlieb in attendance.

I am delighted that my esteemed colleagues from the Society, Nolan and Dr. Mallampalli, both came to work at HealthyWomen once I joined that team. With Battaglino's leadership and her staff, HealthyWomen has continued to educate women on their health and support research into sex differences and now works to encourage policy initiatives furthering women's health.

HealthyWomen has spearheaded in-depth investigations, led by Dr. Mallampalli (now the executive director at the Alliance of Sleep Apnea Partners), on sex differences in the etiology and treatment of chronic pain, COVID-19, migraine disease and the efficacy of biosimilars in men versus women.

Martha Nolan, as HealthyWomen's senior policy advisor, is instrumental in directing HealthyWomen's engagement in policy and in building and strengthening its relationships with federal agencies, healthcare and insurance companies and academia, while promoting improvements in the health of women through research.

HealthyWomen is now a preeminent women's health organization that focuses not on a single condition but on all of women's health and sex and gender differences.

Unfortunately, sex and gender myths and prejudices still degrade the diagnosis and treatment of women. A survey conducted in early 2019 for the *Today* show found that "52% of women, but just 36% of men, say gender discrimination towards patients is a serious problem in the healthcare system." The survey also found that "17% of women but just 6% of men say they have personally been treated differently by a health care provider because of their gender." In addition, "women are more likely than men to say 'a health care provider ignored or dismissed my symptoms' (21% vs. 14%)."[12]

Plus, over the last decade, state and federal legislation has throttled funding for Planned Parenthood, restricting access to wellness care, contraception, cancer screenings, testing for and treatment of sexually transmitted diseases and annual checkups. Now, post *Roe v. Wade*'s defeat in the Supreme Court, political and cultural forces have been unleashed that are threatening not only abortion access—regardless of the circumstances surrounding the pregnancy—but access to contraception. These are just the most obvious instances of how ingrained prejudice against women is in our society and in many parts of the medical community.

Sabra Klein, PhD, professor of molecular microbiology and immunology, director of the Klein Lab and co-director of the Center for

Women's Health, Sex and Gender Research at Johns Hopkins, remains on the front lines of this effort. She told me,

> Here at Hopkins, there's the Specialized Center of Research Excellence (SCORE) on Sex Differences. I am the PI, and we are really very involved in looking at the influence of age and sex in humans and animals [immune response to viral infections and vaccination]. But in general, do I think we are where we should be? In truth, I feel frustration. While I exist in the women's health world, I have to go get my funding and present my research in the infectious disease world, and they are not as open to the idea of sex differences. There's still a lot I have to do to convince people, but this makes me work harder to ensure that we have convincing evidence.

Few healthcare professionals think intentional discrimination is at play here. Instead, it's the vestiges of ingrained gender and sex biases, disproved beliefs and outdated conventions. As Dr. Clayton explained to Duke Health in 2020, "The origins of this situation go back many years."[13] She also proffered that ignorance of sex differences stems from the fact that medical researchers and clinicians have only considered sexual and reproductive function when thinking about what makes men and women distinct, and most lab studies have been done on male cells and animals. "This is a major root of this issue," she concluded.

I'll leave you with these thoughts: In 2020, a United Nations report found that close to 90% of all people hold some form of gender bias against women.[14] A 2018 German study found that doctors often view men with chronic pain as "brave" or "stoic," but women with chronic pain are characterized as being "emotional" or "hysterical."[15] The widespread inequity in medical research perpetuates sex and gender bias. Let's look at the big picture.

## CODA: HIGHLIGHTS FROM 1980 THROUGH 1999

**1980**

- The concept of "hysterical neurosis" was deleted from the American Psychiatric Association's *Diagnostic and Statistical Manual of Mental Disorders.*

**1983**

- The HHS assistant secretary for health appointed the first-ever task force to identify female health issues and an action plan on female health. The task force morphed into HHS's Coordinating Committee on Women's Health in 1984.

**1985**

- The Public Health Service Task Force on Women's Health Issues report came out encouraging a reexamination of current policies about studying women's biology. The report led the National Institutes of Health (NIH) and the Food and Drug Administration (FDA) to issue new guidelines to encourage the inclusion of females in research.

**1989**

- A "Memorandum on Inclusion" from the NIH stated that if females and minorities were excluded from research proposals, scientists should provide a rationale. It was not a mandate, and as a result, not much changed.

**1990**

- The Society for Women's Health Research (SWHR) was founded by Dr. Florence Haseltine.

- A Government Accountability Office (GAO) report, "National Institutes of Health: Problems in Implementing Policy on Women in Study Populations," revealed that women are not sufficiently represented in NIH-funded research.[1]
- A month after the release of the GAO report, the NIH revised its policy to require "a clear rationale" for the exclusion of women and minorities in grant applications for clinical research.
- The NIH established the Office of Research on Women's Health.
- The Women's Health Equity Act, which aimed to promote sex-appropriate healthcare through research and improved access to healthcare services, was introduced in Congress by Senator Barbara Mikulski (D-MD). The act did not pass, despite being co-sponsored by 14 Democrats. That same year Senator Mikulski jump-started the NIH's Office of Research on Women's Health, getting the first funding approved.

## 1991

- HHS established the Office on Women's Health.
- The Office on Women's Health published an *Action Plan for Women's Health* calling for the identification of the health needs of women.

## 1992

- SWHR premieres the *Journal of Women's Health.*
- A GAO report, "Women's Health: FDA Needs to Ensure More Study of Gender Differences in Prescription Drug Testing," says that women are underrepresented in drug trials.[2]

- SWHR asks the GAO to take a look at whether the FDA is examining information on women's responses to drugs before approving medications.

## 1993

- President Clinton signed the NIH Revitalization Act, which mandated that women and minorities be included in all NIH-funded clinical research and phase 3 clinical trials be analyzed for sex differences.
- The FDA throws out its guidelines that banned women with "childbearing potential" from being included in phase 1 and 2 clinical trials.

## 1994

- A congressional mandate created the FDA's Office of Women's Health, largely based on the efforts of SWHR.

## 1995

- The Institute of Medicine (IOM), with SWHR as a partner, submitted a proposal to Congress to write a report on the inclusion of sex differences in medical research, or lack thereof.
- SWHR hosted its fifth Scientific Advisory Meeting (SAM), "Gender-Based Biology: What Does It Mean and Why Does It Matter?"

## 1996

- SWHR hosted its sixth SAM, on the role of sex-based research in human genetics.

- The Institute of Medicine submitted the final proposal to Congress to get funding for *Exploring the Biological Contributions to Human Health: Does Sex Matter?*

**1997**

- SWHR hosted its seventh SAM, exploring sex differences in healthcare delivery outcomes.

**1998**

- SWHR hosted its eighth SAM, looking at sex differences in neurology, psychiatry, immunology and pharmacology.

**1999**

- SWHR published "The Sexual Revolution in Science: What Gender-Based Research Is Telling Us," in the *Journal of Investigative Medicine.*

## PART 2

# Women's Bodies, Women's Voices

This section of the book takes a closer look at the repercussions of sex bias in the lab and in clinical studies and the specific health issues that afflict women because of a lack of understanding of the biological, social, demographic and cultural forces that shape the development and progress of certain diseases.

First, I explore the oversights that have made women's cardiovascular health poorly diagnosed and treated. Then I wade into a neurological stew of issues confronting women who are dealing with conditions that affect the brain, such as chronic pain, migraine and addiction.

After that, I discuss two important female mental health issues, depression and anxiety, before I move on to issues that affect women exclusively: pregnancy, endometriosis, fibroids and menopause.

Disorders and diseases that affect women far more than men are the next area: autoimmune diseases and differences in the immune system's response to infection, Alzheimer's disease, urinary tract issues, irritable bowel syndrome and inflammatory bowel disease, osteoporosis and thyroid diseases. And I look at breast cancer; here, men are in need of more attention, since they are, when affected, almost always diagnosed in a late stage.

I wrap up with a chapter that explores how ignorance of females' unique biology affects the risks and benefits of devices for health management, such as pacemakers and valve replacements.

Throughout these factual explorations there is another layer of information that is especially important. After all, the extraordinary struggle to get the medical research and clinical treatment communities to pay attention to the health of women of all ages and orientations isn't simply the story of institutional resistance to change, government confusion about how to change and corporate focus on bottom lines instead of health outcomes.

It is built upon the tales of individual women who have had to fight to have their health problems acknowledged and treated properly. Many of them have graciously agreed to share their stories.

## CHAPTER 5

# The Big Picture

## Why Sex, Gender and Social Determinants of Health Matter

Knowledge rests not upon truth alone, but upon error also.

—*Carl Jung*

f Carl Jung were right, given the errors that have been made in women's health and in researching the factors that create health inequity, the medical research and clinical care communities should be pretty knowledgeable by now. But they're not. Not as much as they should be.

While corporate and academic research is dragging itself into a more sex-, gender- and race-aware era concerning risk assessment, diagnostic approaches, treatments, medications and devices, much remains to be done to make lab-based and clinical research and clinical practice truly open to sex, gender and race differences.

"What frustrates me," says Virginia Miller, MBA, PhD, professor emeritus of surgery and physiology, former director of the Women's Health Research Center at Mayo Clinic and an early supporter of the Society, "is that when you are in a medical institution with very smart people and scientists, the whole idea of sex as a basic determinant of research seems to go over their heads. It is almost like the opposite of racism. The bias is that there is no difference between the sexes. And since the 2015 NIH mandate, fewer than 60 percent of research studies are fully looking at and reporting sex differences."

## HOW THE SHORTCOMINGS ARE REFLECTED IN LAB STUDIES

In 2016, a study found that only about 31% of write-ups of biomedical experiments mentioned sex or sex differences. And only around 50% of the studies that mentioned sex included both males and females in their study population.[1] That was the same year that the NIH finally issued a regulation requiring—not just suggesting—that sex be included in research design and analysis in studies of vertebrate animals and humans. According to the NIH's "4 Cs of Studying Sex to Strengthen Science," researchers should:

Consider: Design studies that take sex into account or explain why it isn't.

Collect: Gather sex-based data.

Characterize: Analyze sex-based data.

Communicate: Report and publish sex-based data.

What's happened since then? Far too little.

Following the NIH's policy change mandating the consideration of sex as a biological variable in preclinical research, an examination of 2,928 primary research articles published in 2016 in six American Society for Microbiology journals stated that "for animal studies (i.e., studies with any nonhuman vertebrate hosts), most published papers either did not report the sex of the animals or used only female animals, and a minority used only males or both sexes. For published studies using primary cells from diverse animal species (i.e., humans and nonhuman vertebrates), almost all studies failed to report the sex of donors from which the cells were isolated."[2]

In 2020, the authors of a five-year review of progress since the regulation went into effect "called on NIH's various stakeholders to redouble their efforts to integrate SABV [sex as a biological variable] throughout the biomedical research enterprise."[3] They reminded researchers that "sex- and gender-aware investigations are critical to the conduct of rigorous and transparent science and the advancement of personalized medicine."

The persistent lack of transparency in lab results makes it difficult to reproduce experiments in which sex variables affect experimental results. It also makes females and males vulnerable to faulty research conclusions and mistaken medical practices.

There are centers that are doing remarkable lab work, however. At the Klein Laboratory and the Specialized Center of Research Excellence (SCORE) on Sex Differences at Johns Hopkins, Dr. Sabra Klein is doing a deep dive into sex-related responses to the flu vaccine. "We focused on flu vaccines because it was the only vaccine you get every year," Dr. Klein told me.

At Georgetown's Center for the Study of Sex Differences in Health, Aging and Disease, Dr. Kathryn Sandberg is focused on women and cardiovascular diseases. "We investigate why male and female hearts respond differently to very low-calorie diets using experimental animal models. We have seen significant sex differences in the frequency of cardiac arrhythmias after an ischemic event. In that instance, females need more medication to prevent the arrhythmias than males, whereas in models of kidney disease, we have seen that males have more need for medication to protect their kidneys than females."

Everyone benefits when lab-based studies look for significant sex-differences in disease severity and responses to treatment.

## SEX AND GENDER IN THE LAB

Assuming that sex and gender are binary traits determined genetically before birth and consistent throughout life—as is often done when researchers are looking at fruit flies, mice or roundworms (all lab favorites)—obliterates information that sex determination and gender identity can change depending on environmental factors (culture, family, social norms, toxins and outside influences that create epigenetic changes) and differences between groups in basic biology.

What happens to fruit flies and other lab species is frequently generalized to apply to humans—although responsible investigators do wait for confirmation by clinical trials. But still, it slants assumptions and influences the direction of research in clinical settings.

In addition, the influence of environment on gender expression in the lab and in humans has barely been explored, and there's every reason to think that, once investigated, it will reveal important effects on health.

One lab-based study that looked at the impact of climate change on sex and gender determination found that "understanding sex-based responses to climate change allows better modeling of demographic change among marine organisms and the downstream effects for humans.[4]

## HOW SHORTCOMINGS ARE REFLECTED IN CLINICAL TRIALS AND PRACTICE

The negative repercussions of lumping together or failing to look at sex differences in data also appear vividly in human clinical trials and practice. Yet they persist.

You can feel the intense frustration that scientists who are dedicated to acknowledging sex differences experience, even when they're writing for the most staid academic journals.

Nicole Woitowich, PhD, and Teresa Woodruff, PhD, from the Feinberg School of Medicine at Northwestern University, wrote in a 2019 article in the *Proceedings of the National Academy of Science,*

Twenty-five years ago, the National Institutes of Health (NIH) Revitalization Act of 1993 mandated the inclusion of women in clinical research, following decades of misconceptions surrounding women's health and reversing previous guidelines preventing women of childbearing age from participating in early-stage research. Many of us held tight to the belief that this requirement would usher in a new era of discovery where consideration of the female sex would become routine experimental practice both in the clinical and basic sciences.

Yet today, 25 years later, women remain underrepresented as research subjects in the design and development of novel therapeutics and technologies. Moreover, when women are included in NIH-funded clinical research, there is often no attempt to desegregate or analyze data by sex or gender, hindering reproducibility and limiting the potential for sex-specific discoveries and our knowledge about the influences of sex or gender on health and disease.[5]

An examination of progress by Drs. Woitowich, Woodruff and Annaliese Beery, sees the same shortfall. Their 2020 meta-analysis, "A 10-Year Follow-Up Study of Sex Inclusion in the Biological Sciences," found the impact of this policy change on eight of nine biological disciplines—general biology, immunology, neuroscience, physiology, pharmacology, reproduction, endocrinology, behavioral psychology and behavior—was virtually nil.[6] There was no change in the proportion of studies that included data analyzed by sex.

Another interesting study, by researchers at Emory University in 2021, also looked at reporting and misreporting of sex differences. Examining recently published articles for reports about sex differences and non-differences in nine biological disciplines, they found "statistical evidence supporting those differences was often missing. For example, when a sex-specific effect of a manipulation was claimed, authors usually had not tested statistically whether females and males responded differently. Thus, sex-specific effects may be over-reported."[7] They also found that some of the ways studies were done and reported masked sex differences because the sexes were pooled without first testing for a difference. Their conclusion, which I applaud, is that there's a "need for continuing efforts to train researchers [on] how to test for and report sex differences in order to promote rigor and reproducibility in biomedical research."

As Martha Nolan, HealthyWomen's senior policy advisor, points out, "Although getting more women into clinical trials is important, it is only part of the battle. Just including women in equal numbers doesn't matter if you're not analyzing for differences. Who benefited? Who got hurt? Was it equal among subgroups, or was one outcome more predominant among men or women? Drilling down in the data is crucial."

Lack of financial support for clinical studies that include or focus on women's health is an obstacle to progress. A 2021 study by Art Mirin, PhD, in the *Journal of Women's Health* concluded: "We find that in nearly three-quarters of the cases where a disease afflicts primarily one gender, the funding pattern favors males, in that either the disease affects more women and is underfunded (with respect to burden), or the disease affects more men and is overfunded. Moreover, the disparity between actual funding and that which is commensurate with burden is nearly twice as large for diseases that favor males versus those that favor females." In other words, says Dr. Mirin, "the NIH applies a disproportionate share of its resources to diseases that affect primarily men, at the expense of those that affect primarily women."[8]

Evaluations that are made day-to-day in doctors' offices remain in large part the product of completely or mostly male-centered research, as well as un-researched assumptions about sex, gender and race. Just how many mistakes this causes in the diagnosis and treatment of women's conditions is impossible to estimate—but you can bet it is huge. So, let's take a brief look at how sex, race and gender get short shrift in doctors' offices across the country.

## HARD TO SWALLOW

Many medications cause women problems that were never looked for or anticipated. This is because there are many factors in female biology that impact how a particular medication works or doesn't work. Extra body fat can change absorption; so can sex differences in digestion. For example, men produce more gastric acid than women. As a result, if women take medications, like the antifungal ketoconazole, that need an acidic environment to be absorbed, they may not get the full dose required for effective treatment. Women also move food through their digestive tract more slowly than men do—so medications they are supposed to take on an empty stomach (certain antibiotics) may in fact encounter undigested food that blocks their effectiveness. Hormones, of course, play a major role in how drugs are metabolized, and since women's hormones fluctuate during their menstrual cycle and during perimenopause, that can affect how a woman's liver breaks down and clears a medication. None of these factors are taken into consideration in the prescription of most medicines.

No wonder eight out of ten of the drugs removed from the US market between 1997 and 2000 were withdrawn because of side effects that occurred mainly or exclusively in women. From 2004 through

2013, women in the United States experienced more than 2 million drug-related adverse events, compared with 1.3 million for men.[9]

The classic case of how badly things can turn out when women are not part of the evaluation process for medications is Ambien, says Alyson J. McGregor, MD, MA, associate dean for faculty affairs and development at the University of South Carolina School of Medicine, Greenville, co-founder of the Sex and Gender Women's Health Collaborative at the Warren Alpert Medical School of Brown University and a member of the NIH Advisory Committee on Research on Women's Health. "The drug was released into the market 25 years ago and was prescribed for 20 years, mostly to women. There were almost 1,000 reports of women experiencing impaired driving the morning after taking it," says Dr. McGregor. It was a worst-case scenario for post-market surveillance.

That prompted the drug company to launch another study on a similar formulation of the medication. The researchers gave the drug to men and women and after four hours put them into a simulated driving experiment. Women were crashing cars, men were not. It turned out females had two times the serum concentration of the drug as males after equal lengths of time.

"There were real consequences—and the injuries and human toll from Ambien mis-prescribing could have been avoided if they'd had the sex-specific data to begin with," adds Dr. McGregor. Eventually, the Food and Drug Administration (FDA) created its first-ever sex-based dosage guidelines—for Ambien.

While Ambien cleared at a much slower rate in females than males, the opposite turned out to be the case (also discovered post-marketing) for the anti-seizure drug lamotrigine when taken by pregnant women. Fully 77% of females had a more than 10 times higher rate of clearance while pregnant compared to before they became pregnant, putting them at a much higher risk for seizures.[10]

## WHAT DO WE KNOW?

A 2001 Government Accountability Office report, sponsored by Senators Tom Harkin, Olympia Snowe and Barbara Mikulski and Representative Henry Waxman, was the first glimpse at the treatment problems that arise when women are not included in studies for medications.[11] The report found that eight of ten medications withdrawn from circulation between 1997 and 2001 posed greater health risks for women than for men. Four were taken mostly by women, so that may account for the increased problems; four clearly posed more health risks for women than men; and two were found to be almost equally risky for men and women, although one did belong to a class of drugs known to pose greater risks for women.

Even today, there is a deficit in understanding about the right medications to use and dosages of meds that are effective and safe for women. A 2018 study in the *British Journal of Pharmacology* reported that while there is often a gender balance in phase 2 and 3 trials, in phase 1 trials, women represent only 22% of participants.[12] The researchers went on to conclude that "when compared with US disease prevalence data, 10 drugs (26%) had a greater than 20% difference between the proportion of females affected with the disease compared with representation in clinical trials." Put another way: Even when researchers were looking at medications being developed to treat diseases that affect more women than men, there were not many women participating in those clinical trials.

As recently as 2020, a meta study of several thousand medical journal articles revealed what the researchers called a "drug dose gender gap" for 86 FDA-approved medications, such as antidepressants, cardiovascular drugs, anti-seizure drugs and pain meds.[13] When women were given the same dose of a medication as men, they experienced higher concentrations of the drug in their blood and it took longer to clear. Overall, they had almost twice as many adverse drug reactions as men—including nausea, headache, depression, cognitive deficits, seizures, hallucinations, agitation and cardiac anomalies.[14]

In the beginning of 2023, the nonprofit Bioethics International published a new pharma scorecard in *BMJ Medicine*.[15] The scorecard includes evaluation of inclusion and transparency in clinical trials concerning participation of men and women, various ethnic groups and people who are older.

The researchers found that in 64 trials of novel cancer therapeutics conducted by 25 pharma companies from 2010 to 2017, 56% of the companies included adequate numbers of women, 25% adequately included older adults, but just 16% adequately represented patients who were not white and no companies adequately represented Hispanic patients. Only half of the companies included an adequate number of Asian participants. Only one company, United Therapeutics, received a perfect score.

## A POSITIVE EXAMPLE

Bringing sex into a clinical study can have startlingly beneficial—and illuminating—consequences: Naltrexone is an oral form of Narcan (naloxone), and when researchers wanted to see if it could help men and women decrease cocaine and alcohol use, they were in for a surprise. In a 2007 study, researchers found that 150 mg a day of naltrexone, when combined with psychosocial treatment for 12 weeks, reduced cocaine and alcohol use in men, but in women it was associated with higher rates of use, as well as a more severe impact of addiction on daily life.[16]

As an aside, it's often said that it is too expensive, difficult or in- convenient to disaggregate information on females in study results.

But researchers who care have looked at these objections and found that making experiment designs more efficient can eliminate much of that burden. They estimate that sample sizes may need to be increased by 14–33% to account for the extra parameter being estimated, but they do not need to be doubled.[17] And the rewards in depth of understanding and improved efficacy of medications, for example, offer savings in the long run.

## REFINING SEX DIFFERENCES BY LOOKING AT SUBGROUPS: WHAT'S SMART, WHAT'S NOT

While it is of enormous importance that females/women and males/men be considered in the full range of research and data analysis, it is equally important that subgroups of females and women be accurately brought into research as well.

"We have to define that women are not homogeneous," says Dr. Nanette Wenger. "There are subgroups . . . racial and ethnic minorities. And we need to define the particular problems for these women—the doubly disadvantaged and elderly who are excluded." The four steps Dr. Wenger says are needed to improve care for all women are: investigate, educate (by translating research to the clinical community), advocate and legislate.

Currently, that is an evolving process, and many questions remain about the nature of racial/ethnic differences in healthcare experiences and in prevalence and/or manifestation of various disorders.

I suggest that a lot of the confusion about making distinctions between females who are Caucasian, African, African American, Hispanic, American Indian, and so on, might be best addressed by abandoning the question of whether or not to use race in medical evaluations and asking instead, "How can we use race wisely?"

We know we use it badly; so much that is currently done in the name of race recognition is tainted by unconscious, inadvertent, intentional and/or systemic racism.

Over and over in research papers we find that female study subjects are willy-nilly categorized as Black/non-Black, white/nonwhite, Caucasian, African American, et cetera. American Indians are also lumped together. Jennifer Tsai, a writer for *Scientific American,* brings up a profound point in her article "What Role Should Race Play in Medicine?"[18] She writes that researchers lump more than 500 separate tribes living across a vast stretch of geography into the racial category "American Indian." We don't make "European" a racial category, she says, so why do we do it to American Indians?

To see how this plays out in the actual practice of medicine, let's look at the FRAX tool.[19] Its goal is to evaluate osteoporosis and bone fracture risk of patients (mostly women). It was developed by studying population-based cohorts from Europe, North America, Asia and Australia. The site says, "It is based on individual patient models that integrate the risks associated with clinical risk factors as well as bone mineral density (BMD) at the femoral neck." The US version is the only one of 72 versions to divide populations into four "races": Caucasian, Black, Hispanic and Asian.

Questions arise: When using FRAX, if a US doctor has a Chinese patient, is she the same as an Asian American female in terms of risk calculation? In an Asian version of FRAX there are 11 divisions for various groups, but in the United States all Asians are in one group. How does that make any scientific sense? And Hispanics? A huge, diverse group—not a race—and yet all in one group in FRAX. So how does that work?

For the Hispanic/Latino community, long-held assumptions based on demographic data get blown away when health and sickness are accurately evaluated. "The biggest issue," says Jane L. Delgado, PhD, president and CEO of the National Alliance for Hispanic Health, "is that researchers are reluctant to change the conceptual frameworks they use regardless of the emerging evidence."

For example, if lower income alone were the major cause of poor health, then Hispanics, who have less income than other groups, should have terrible health. However, Hispanics have a longer life expectancy (77.7 years) than non-Hispanic whites (76.4 years) and non-Hispanic Blacks (70.8 years).

"Hispanics are an afterthought," says Dr. Delgado, "which is unacceptable, especially given the size of the Hispanic population. We are nearly 63 million, which equals the sum of 100% of all African Americans (40.1 million) plus 86% of all Asian Americans (20.3 million). And clustering Black and Hispanic women together, which often happens, is not only scientifically not helpful, it also diminishes the issues and values of each community."

### ARTIFICIAL INTELLIGENCE NEGLIGENCE

Gender, along with sex, is often overlooked or mistakenly parsed when examining female/women's health issues. Even when there is new diagnostic technology available, such as AI, it may fall far short. As a 2020 study in *Nature,* "Sex and Gender Differences and Biases in Artificial Intelligence for Biomedicine and Healthcare," points out, "The design of the majority of algorithms ignore the sex and gender dimension and its contribution to health and disease differences among individuals. Failure in accounting for these differences will generate sub-optimal results and produce mistakes as well as discriminatory outcomes."[20]

Marjorie Jenkins, MD, former director of medical initiatives and scientific engagement in the FDA's Office of Women's Health, currently associate provost and dean of the University of South Carolina School of Medicine, Greenville, told me: "If you use artificial intelligence in healthcare, too often it uses data that is already out there, which is biased, and then there's a ripple effect—you create an algorithm that's biased too." She says: "It's because eons ago, scientists decided to ignore two basic human variables which we all have without fail—sex and gender."

## WHERE DO WE GO FROM HERE?

It's true that sex and gender can each separately affect health and health outcomes. But usually they are intertwined. Biological sex is more likely to be related to how disease occurs and develops. Gender may have a significant impact on the manifestation and reporting of symptoms and on healthcare providers' recognition of symptoms.[21] Gender also influences treatment recommendations and options and affects what kind of care is made available and its quality.

Social determinants of health have a significant impact on many women. Mayo Clinic's special report, *Race and Health,* says social determinants of health include economic stability, education, healthcare, one's neighborhood and built environment and social and community context.[22]

- Economic stability is impacted by poverty, employment, food insecurity and housing instability.
- Educational determinants are high school graduation, enrollment in higher education, language and literacy and early childhood education and development.

- Healthcare issues include access to primary care, access to health services and health literacy.

- Neighborhood and built environment covers access to healthy foods, quality of housing, crime and violence and environmental conditions.

- Social and community context ranges from social cohesion and civic participation to discrimination and incarceration.

That's why it's important to make the public, the government, research institutions and academics, as well as physicians, aware of the specific health issues that require (but do not have) a full understanding of the sex, demographic and gender distinctions that impact the incidence, diagnosis and treatment of diseases and disorders.

## SEX- AND GENDER-RELATED DISTINCTIONS

The areas that create distinct health issues—among different groups of women and between women and men—include genetics, epigenetics, hormones, immune function, aging and neurocognitive decline and response to medications.[23]

- In the field of genetics, we know that sex chromosomes primarily determine differences in sex organs and resulting expression of sex steroids (they influence sexual dimorphism and bone growth and remodeling). But we also know that the X chromosome contains regions that produce distinct differences in males and females in many organ systems— not just in reproductive organs. Research is only beginning to understand how complex the X chromosome is and how it creates differences in autosomal expression (where just one mutation of a gene causes a different manifestation of a trait or a disease).

- Epigenetics, or changes in gene expression, may happen because of a number of factors, from environmental toxins and stress to hormones, enzymes and even DNA. Sociocultural gender differences in diet and exercise, cigarette smoking or social pressures can also trigger differing gene expressions in women. On top of that, there are sex differences in the mechanics of epigenetic functions. That is seen in differences in how external and internal influences can alter genetic expression.

- Frequently, sex differences, as well as expressions of gender, result from the hormone soup that flows through the body. Hormones trigger a specific ordering of cells in a fetus and are linked to a wide range of sex-specific conditions and disorders. They are implicated in the prevalence in females of autoimmune disorders, osteoporosis, some cardiometabolic disorders and, according to preliminary research, perhaps Alzheimer's disease.

- Research also indicates that immune function differs between men and women.[24] For example, some vaccines have higher efficacy in premenopausal women. Sex also influences transplant rejection and it is thought that fluctuating hormones may explain why autoimmune conditions are more common in women. Alzheimer's, which research now indicates may have an autoimmune component, is almost twice as common in women as men, and, according to Harvard Medical School, that's not just because of a longer life span.[25]

- Other cognition problems that affect women also may be the result of age-related decline in estradiol, and metabolic disruptions are involved. One complex sex–disease interaction is seen in the relationship of type 2 diabetes to dementia. For women, type 2 diabetes increases dementia risk by 60%, and the risk for dementia in women with diabetes is 19% greater than for men with diabetes.[26]

## SEX, GENDER AND RACE IN INTERACTIONS WITH THE HEALTHCARE SYSTEM

The way healthcare is delivered and the outcomes of treatment are directly affected by discrimination because of sex, gender, race/ethnicity, sexuality and socioeconomic status.

Less than half of US adults get health insurance through work; 44% of men enjoy that perk, but just 35% of women do.[27] In 2020 among those with work-based insurance, 6% of women and 3% of men found medical care unaffordable. In addition, 8.1% of women and 5.4% of men said dental care was priced out of range, 5.2% of women and 2.7% of men said prescription medications were unaffordable and 2.1% of women and 0.8% of men reported that they could not afford mental health care.[28]

For those who don't have work-based insurance the situation is far tougher. KFF reports that around 40% of American women and men have postponed getting medical care or skipped it altogether because they cannot afford it.[29]

## HEARTLESS MEDICAL CARE

The uninsured or underinsured face daunting challenges when it comes to getting proper care. Florence Champagne is chairperson and CEO of the Open My Heart Foundation, which is dedicated to helping eliminate heart health disparities among African American women and women of color, and a spokesperson for WomenHeart, a national coalition of women who support women living with or who are at risk of heart disease. She recalls that, without insurance, she battled to get a proper diagnosis for her ever-worsening heart condition that led to a heart attack in 2012—followed by emergency open heart surgery:

> The first time I went to the ER it was because I wasn't feeling right—I had a sensation in my jaw and shortness of breath. Periodically, it would feel like tiny stabs of pain in my chest, as if someone was poking or stabbing me with a knife. It would come and go. I had shrugged it off until I knew it was not natural to feel this way.
>
> But all the woman at the ER's intake desk was interested in was whether I had insurance. And I didn't. I was between jobs. Also, I learned later that I didn't present symptoms as if I were suffering a classic heart attack. She said, "You look fine. You're relatively young, and don't look like anything is wrong with you!" During one ER visit I was told to seek counseling, as if the pain was all in my head. I felt unworthy of getting any help and at a disadvantage right from the start.
>
> I kept going back to the ER—I must have gone to the ER six times over the course of a year—because I was getting worse. Each time my blood pressure was elevated. The doctor would send me home with medications for high blood pressure. Eventually I was told that I had an enlarged heart and angina. "Take the pills when you feel pain and go away," was the message.
>
> Sometime later I met a cardiologist. He reviewed my records and asked why I hadn't had a cardiac catheterization. I didn't even know what that was! He explained to me that it's when they inject dye in your system to see if there is any blockage. He then asked me what type of insurance I had. I told him that I didn't have any.

It was as if a light bulb went off. He said, "That's why you haven't had the proper diagnostic testing! Don't worry, I'll find a way to get the test for you."

As I waited for the cardiologist to get back to me, I went about my business. Approximately one week later, I dropped to my knees one day in the lobby of a public building. I couldn't breathe. . . . I started sweating profusely and pain started radiating down my arm. I knew this was more serious than the other times. I said a simple prayer, "God, please don't let me die like this." That's when the doctors found that I had a 99.9% blockage in my main artery—and I had emergency open heart surgery.

If you are uninsured, or even underinsured, and you don't have anyone fighting for you, this is the way you get treated. I nearly lost my life because of the misdiagnosis, delay in treatment, being told "you look fine," and quite simply, inequities in treatment. As a social worker and advocate for others, I now had to advocate for myself.

This experience allowed me to spread the word about the obstacles we face as women when we don't present the same symptoms as men. Now my mission is making sure women of color are aware of heart disease symptoms, stressing the importance of being your own best advocate, and pushing until you get the help. I also make sure they are aware of the importance of having someone go with you to the ER or the doctor's office to help you ask the right questions and stand up for yourself.

## OTHER OBSTACLES

### A Failure to Communicate

Once they are interacting with the healthcare system, women may encounter obstacles to treatment because of patient–healthcare provider communication problems that are influenced by the gender and race of the physician and the patient.[30] This results in women's increased disease burden and differences in treatment.

### Systemic Racism

Women of color, particularly African Americans, pay a tremendous price for the systemic ignorance of the biological and environmental factors that impact their health and healthcare. "Black women and white women in the United States lead very different lives—economically, socially, geographically," says Linda Goler Blount, MPH, president and CEO of Black Women's Health Imperative. "And those differences affect their health, but apparently not any of the official recommendations about their health."

According to the Susan G. Komen Foundation, overall, the incidence of breast cancer is slightly lower among Black women than white women. But death from breast cancer is greater in Black women; in fact, from 2012 to 2016, it was around 40% higher in Black than white women.

Some contributing factors have to do with social environment, racism, chronic stress and increased rates of obesity and chronic inflammation, and some have to do with biological differences that help shape the development of diseases and reactions to medications and treatments. These issues are only beginning to be guessed at or considered in making treatment choices.

## GENDER NONCONFORMING AND TRANSGENDER BIAS

The transgender community also pays a big price for systemic medical ignorance. If a patient is transgender or nonconforming, they/he/she very often experiences microaggression or flat-out discrimination. For

transgender women (male at birth and identifying as female) or transgender men (female at birth and identifying as male), this can lead to
avoidance of healthcare—and worse health outcomes.

A 2021 fact sheet from the Center for American Progress revealed
that almost half of transgender adults say they have experienced mis-
treatment or discrimination when dealing with a healthcare provider,
and just under 20% say they had been refused care because they were
transgender or gender nonconforming. In addition, 40% said they
postponed care, even if injured or sick, because of discrimination and
disrespect.[31]

The unmet—but often more prevalent—conditions that affect the
LGBTQ+ community include behavioral and mental health problems,
such as mood disorders and anxiety, eating disorders, alcohol and
substance abuse, tobacco use and suicide.[32] Physical issues that affect
the LGBTQ+ community more than the general population include
HIV/AIDS,[33] obesity (lesbian and bisexual women) and breast cancer
(a study in the Netherlands found that trans women have a 46 times
greater risk of developing breast cancer than cis men do).[34] LGBTQ+
people also experience higher rates of HPV infection and related cervical or anal cancers.[35] In addition, older members of the community
report that they have more chronic conditions than other groups and
less social support.[36]

## DISINTEREST IN WOMEN'S SEXUALITY AND
## REPRODUCTIVE/GENITAL ORGANS

There is an odd combination of overfocus on the women-only aspects of
health, pregnancy, menstruation, and so on—what Dr. Wenger called
"bikini medicine"—and a willful disregard for women-specific biology.

Take the clitoris—a sexual organ about which almost nothing is truly known and there is very little research. One 2019 study that explored the literature found that in a clinical setting, most doctors (even gynos) don't examine the vulva and clitoris and, as a consequence, frequently miss sexual health conditions such as clitoral adhesions.[37]

Lack of knowledge about the structure and function of the clitoris can also lead to secondary postoperative damage that leaves women without the ability to orgasm, according to Helen O'Connell, MD, a research professor at Australia's Monash University. In 2005, she published a comprehensive study showing that the outer clitoris—the part that can be seen and touched—was like the tip of the penis.[38] The clitoris in fact extends below the surface and is made up of two teardrop-shaped bulbs, two arms and a shaft.

"You always need to be thinking of what's underneath, what's hidden from view that you're potentially altering" when doing urethral or pelvic mesh surgeries, cautions Dr. O'Connell.[39]

We are living through the #MeToo movement, and there is a growing recognition of how frequently women are victims of sexual violence and assault. #MeToo in women's health is still unfolding, and while many advances have occurred in the last 25 years, we are not done yet. The story, or should I say journey, of equal treatment and understanding sex and gender differences in prevention, diagnosis and treatment is incomplete.

That's my overview of the current situation and the issues confronting women and the healthcare system. Now let's look at why sex matters in terms of specific health challenges.

# CHAPTER 6

# The Heart of the Matter

## What Happens to Women's Cardio Health When Sex Is Ignored

All the research on heart disease has really been based on
men, and needs to be updated with research on women—
even very early stage research is done using male rats!

—*Laura Bush, founder of the Laura W. Bush*
*Institute for Women's Health*[1]

For all of us who spend our lives fighting for inclusion of women in clinical trials and females in research studies, there is nothing more poignant than when we run into someone who is currently battling to get the sex-specific and gender-appropriate care she needs. Instantly, the debates about the unique influence on health and illness of hormones, cellular structures, neurons and organ function shift from being academic considerations to topics that contain palpable human emotion and pain. This stuff matters, every day, in every way, to millions of women.

Let's look at how lack of clarity about how females experience various conditions plays out in women's lives. In this chapter we explore heart disease—the number one killer of women in the United States.[2]

## TAKE IT TO HEART

Heart disease threatens all women.[3] It kills more Black and white women than any other condition. It is tied with cancer as the top-ranking killer among American Indian and Alaska Native women. Among Hispanic, Asian and Pacific Islander women, cancer is the number one killer, but heart disease is a close second. In all, 314,186 women died from heart disease in 2020, accounting for 20% of female deaths. Yet only around 44% of women are aware that heart disease is their number one killer.[4] And the medical community seems to lack sufficient awareness too. Over and over women with heart disease are dismissed, overlooked, undertreated and understudied.

"At every stop along the way we are falling short," says Alexandra Lansky, MD, FESC, FACC, director of the Yale Heart and Vascular Clinical Research Program and the Cardiovascular Research Group. "We don't have enough women cardiologists. Women cardiologists don't have an opportunity to be in leadership positions. Patients don't know the symptoms of heart disease, so they are not coming forward, and when they do come to the ER, their symptoms aren't recognized there either."

## A LONG AND WINDING ROAD

Glenda Sexauer was 47 years old when she started experiencing fatigue and weight gain.

> I was always active. I did a marathon and the MS bike ride that covered 150 miles in two days. So, I was bewildered and went to see several doctors. They suggested it was related to chronic stress, menopause, thyroid disease (I was diagnosed with Hashimoto's, an autoimmune cause of low thyroid function). But it was not until I went with my husband to Hawaii for our twenty-fifth anniversary that I knew that something more was going on. I became so weak I couldn't even walk up two steps.
>
> When we got home I went straight to the doctor and [they] diagnosed me with congestive heart failure, admitted me to the hospital and they removed 30 pounds of fluid through diuretics! I was in heart failure and it had been unidentified and overlooked.
>
> Unfortunately, the day I was to be discharged—thank heavens it took forever to get through all the rigmarole—I went into cardiac arrest in the hospital. They defibrillated my heart and put me into a medically induced coma for four days to give my heart

a chance to rest and start to recover. I had an ICD (a combination of a pacemaker and defibrillator) implanted.

That was about 13 years ago. I am very lucky. These days I work out doing HIIT [high-intensity interval training] four days a week, hike three miles a week, do yoga twice a week and babysit for my grandchildren.

When I think back I realize that each specialist I saw was just thinking about their own field of study—no one imagined someone fit and young like I was could have heart disease. For example, when I thought my symptoms might be related to menopause I went to my gynecologist and all he said was, "Your hormones are fine." He never said that maybe I should get checked by someone else. He wasn't interested in figuring out why I was gaining so much weight and was so fatigued. And until I was almost dying, no one, including me, ever thought it could be from heart problems.

The campaign to have women's heart health studied and treated as a unique entity—acknowledging where it overlaps with men's experience of the condition and where it differs—has been waged for decades.

"I became involved in the push to get females represented in basic research, clinical trials and treatment options because many decades ago, as I treated women who had cardiovascular disease, I searched the databases to find information on women. There was none," says Dr. Nanette Wenger. "That's when I coined the term *bikini medicine*.

"In the 1980s, the information I found about women's health was whatever was covered by a bikini and the rest of the woman was left unstudied. There was a tacit assumption that a 50-year-old white man was the model for cardiovascular health and could be extrapolated to the whole world."

An example of the detrimental effects of not including women in cardiovascular research was the 1989 Physicians' Health Study, which reported that daily low-dose aspirin reduced the risk of a first myocardial infarction by 44%. As a result, physicians started prescribing an aspirin a day as a preventative measure for heart disease to both men and women. But the Physicians' Health Study only included white men. Subsequent research found that for women, daily low-dose aspirin did not reduce the risk of myocardial infarction and could increase the risk of internal bleeding.[5]

To combat the lack of knowledge about women and heart disease, in 2006 and then again in 2011, the Society for Women's Health Research (SWHR) and WomenHeart published "The 10Q Report: Advancing Women's Heart Health Through Improved Research, Diagnosis and Treatment."[6] They identified the top 10 unanswered research questions related to the diagnosis and treatment of heart disease in women that would most impact the cardiovascular health of women and spurred increased attention on the field.

In addition, in 2009, the Society launched the Interdisciplinary Network on Cardiovascular Disease, bringing together eminent cardiovascular researchers and clinicians. It ran from 2009 to 2014.

I am proud that the Society and WomenHeart were able to work with experts like Dr. Wenger and cardiologist and researcher Dr. Sharonne Hayes, founder of the Women's Heart Clinic at Mayo Clinic, to stimulate research on sex and gender differences in heart disease and increase awareness and knowledge of women's heart health issues. We helped create research initiatives on everything from sex and gender differences in heart disease pathophysiology to challenges in healthcare delivery and new treatment approaches that reduced women's cardiovascular disease burden.

But for all that effort, there are still many black holes in the care being offered.

"I see several patients every week who come to me with signs of heart disease that were missed either completely or for too long by their other doctors," says C. Noel Bairey Merz, MD, FACC, director of the Barbra Streisand Women's Heart Center at Cedars-Sinai. "For example, I saw a woman in her midfifties who had been hospitalized after a heart attack. She had an angiogram that revealed nothing and was sent home despite the fact she had continuing chest discomfort. So, she then has another heart attack and survives that too. But it's not until she gets to our clinic and we do noninvasive imaging to measure small artery blood flow that she is diagnosed correctly."

"We are just at the beginning of understanding the difference between the sexes when it comes to heart disease," concludes Dr. Bairey Merz. As a result, she says, we see statistics like these—but no conclusive findings as to why these are the emerging realities about women and heart disease:

- In a meta-analysis of over 850,000 people, the relative risk for cardiovascular disease was 44% greater in women with type 2 diabetes than in men with the disease.[7]
- In the Framingham Heart Study, obesity increased the relative risk of coronary artery disease by 64% in women and 46% in men.[8]
- The ratio of women to men with rheumatoid arthritis is 2.5:1; for lupus it is 9:1. Patients with rheumatoid arthritis have double to triple the risk of heart attack and a 50% higher risk of stroke.[9] For lupus, the risk of heart attack is 9 to 50 times greater than for the general population.

- In women, narrowing arteries (ischemic heart disease [IHD])
  does show up as it does in men, as coronary artery disease
  (CAD) caused by plaque blocking blood flow in the arteries.[10]
  But in women it is also caused by coronary microvascular
  dysfunction (e.g., endothelial dysfunction, abnormal vessel
  dilation and contraction), spontaneous coronary artery
  dissection (SCAD) and stress-induced cardiomyopathy.
  And, studies show, when women show up with male-style
  symptoms of CAD, they are more likely to be diagnosed—
  and then treated—like men.

To highlight the underdiagnosis and undertreatment of women
with IHD, Dr. Bernadine Healy, former NIH director, once called it
the Yentl Syndrome, based on the Barbra Streisand movie in which
she played an Ashkenazi Jewish girl in Poland who decides to dress
and live like a boy so that she can receive an education in Talmudic
law after her father dies.[11] The problem persists today.

"The WISE study,[12] which finally showed that women with heart
disease often have small artery dysfunction, is one example of physiological causes of women's heart conditions being overlooked and
undiagnosed as a result of using male-standard testing," explains Dr.
Bairey Merz.

According to a 2016 study, "Cardiovascular Disease in Women:
Clinical Perspectives," the most important characteristics of IHD in
women are: "(1) a higher prevalence of angina, (2) a lower burden of
obstructive CAD on angiography and (3) a poorer prognosis in com-
parison to men."[13] The study also states that "current risk scores, based
on ACS [acute coronary syndrome] thresholds determined in predom-
inantly male-based samples, do not accurately predict risk in women."

In addition, biomarkers such as proneurotensin are sex-specific and associated with the development of CVD and subsequent heart attacks and stroke only in women, clearly demonstrating the need for more research in this area.[14]

The result of all these slights, oversights and systemic myopia is that, traditionally, women have been less likely to receive cholesterol- and triglyceride-lowering medications, aspirin and guidance about heart-protective lifestyle changes than guys who are diagnosed with a similar atherosclerotic cardiovascular disease risk.[15] And when women do receive appropriate treatment, it is often less aggressive than men's.

One 2008 study in the *Journal of Women's Health,* titled "Disparities in Physicians' Interpretations of Heart Disease Symptoms by Patient Gender: Results of a Video Vignette Factorial Experiment," found that middle-aged women with chest pain and other symptoms of heart disease were twice as likely to be diagnosed with a mental illness as men who had the same symptoms.[16]

In addition, cardiac rehab is less used—women are around half as likely to do cardiac rehab as men—in part because of under-referral by doctors and in part because of lifestyle demands and restrictions that make it difficult.

Lyn Behnke, a cardiovascular nurse practitioner and chair of WomenHeart's board of directors, recalls once asking a cardiologist, "What do you think about nonobstructive coronary artery disease?"

"I asked," says Behnke, "because it is the reason for a lot of missed and mis- diagnoses in women. His response? 'I got rid of those whiny women—you are all middle-aged, fat and whiny.' So, I made it my mission to prove what a problem microvascular disease is."

As Behnke's 2022 paper, "The Danger of Underdiagnosing Coronary Microvascular Disease in Women," published in the *Journal of the American Association of Nurse Practitioners,* states, "Symptomatic patients often are left undiagnosed, frustrated and at risk of adverse cardiac events. Frequently, the only method of diagnosis is treatment of the symptoms."[17]

Just look at the findings from other recent studies on women and heart attacks.

- In the ER, women and people of color under age 55 with chest pain wait longer than white men the same age to be evaluated by a doctor. Plus, women are less likely to be kept under observation or hospitalized than men.[18]

- Heart attack diagnosis is missed in women more often than in men. In 2021 the European Society of Cardiology announced the findings of a 12-year study that "in women, 5% of ACS [acute coronary syndrome] were initially misdiagnosed, whereas in men, 3% of ACS were initially misdiagnosed. After multivariate analysis, female gender was an independent risk factor for an initial impression of non-ACS." Physicians are also more likely in their initial diagnosis to consider ACS the cause of chest pain in men compared to women.[19]

- Women 18 to 55 years old receive less aggressive care than men after a heart attack with pumping failure. They are also more likely to die before being discharged than men the same age.[20]

- Heart attacks in women under the age of 55 are often missed, dismissed or misdiagnosed. In a 2018 study published in *Circulation,* women exhibited substantially more variation in unique symptom phenotypes than men. And those symptoms far too often do not register with healthcare providers as symptoms of a heart attack.[21]

### THE SEARCHING HEART

Mary Anne Norling had a long history of heart-related issues, including preeclampsia when she was pregnant at 23 and a stroke two and a half years later.[22] Then in her fifties, when she was living an active, healthy lifestyle, she suddenly saw her cholesterol bounce up to around 300 despite being on a statin, and she started having arm pain upon exertion. Her internist suggested she get a full cardiology workup.

"Even with all my background of high cholesterol, preeclampsia, history of a stroke—and after the stress echo workup—I was told there was nothing wrong with me," Norling says. Only four months later, while vacationing in Tahoe with her family, Norling suffered a heart attack at age 57.

After her recovery she set out to find a cardiologist she could work with—and who would pay attention to what she had to say. "It's not uncommon that women with heart issues have to see two to three cardiologists until they find somebody who will listen to them," Norling says. "Well, I'm on my third cardiologist. Thank heavens I kept looking. He's wonderful."

The latest insights into differences in the way men and women develop heart disease expose significant reasons that women are so often mis- or underdiagnosed when presenting with heart attacks. Some examples of recently revealed intrinsic differences in the development and manifestation of heart disease:

- Men and women develop heart disease differently, according to a 2020 study that uncovered the fact that different minerals block heart valves in men versus women.[23]
- The same year, research showed that older women generally have many more symptoms of heart attack than men.[24]

• Research from 2021 suggests male-female differences in protein expression occur immediately after embryonic cells become heart cells—and before sex hormones impact an embryo.[25]

## ADDITIONAL COMPLEXITIES

"Take a breath—it's not that simple." That's the message that Dr. Hayes wants to call to women's (and doctors') attention. As Dr. Hayes says:

> The biggest favor we can do for women is to make sure that they receive no ambiguous messages about the fact that chest pain is the number one symptom of heart attack in women, as it is in men. There are very few sex differences in the prevalence of various heart attack symptoms and in fact there are no symptoms that are unique to women.
>
> But I do I think we need to emphasize that women often have multiple symptoms, and women need to be aware that there are less common symptoms such as nausea, vomiting and shortness of breath. Also, there are a couple of additional reasons for delay in diagnosis of heart disease in women. Sometimes a woman may come in with eight symptoms and a man with two—for the same condition. A woman may mention nausea and forget to mention chest pain, for example. That can slow down diagnosis. And sometimes it is a gender difference that interferes—a woman will say, "I was caring for my ailing spouse so I couldn't go to the ER." I have even heard excuses like, "I had to finish cooking dinner."

## BEYOND HEART ATTACKS

Heart attacks aren't the only cardiovascular conditions for which women struggle to obtain a proper diagnosis and timely, effective trcatment. Other conditions include cardiomyopathy, high blood pressure, stroke and SCAD. Heart surgeries, such as coronary bypass, are also often not done on women using the most validated procedures.

## HEART HEALTH FOR THE LONG RUN

Darlene Scott doesn't let heart disease define her. She keeps moving forward; one foot in front of the other. And she wants other women of color to do the same. As she states:

> Women of color are disproportionately affected by the disease, and often don't know what to look for. We have to become more aware of the signs and symptoms of heart disease. And we have to stick up for ourselves, because sometimes heart disease symptoms are mistaken for something else—which is what happened in my case.
>
> I was training for a marathon in 2016 and noticed I was experiencing shortness of breath and fatigue. It felt different than a normal response to training. I thought it was my allergies.
>
> It took a long time until I found out it wasn't asthma. In fact, I had an enlarged heart, also known as cardiomyopathy. But no one had thought to look for that for quite a while.
>
> Within a year I had to have a pacemaker implanted and was also diagnosed with sarcoidosis, an autoimmune disease.
>
> After that I was determined to help other women in the African American community learn about their heart disease risks and the challenges of getting optimal care. I felt like I didn't have anyone to talk to after being diagnosed. Not any more!

## HIGH BLOOD PRESSURE: A SERIOUS RISK FACTOR
## FOR STROKE, HEART ATTACK AND DEMENTIA

Dr. Bairey Merz and colleagues, in a 2020 article in *JAMA Cardiology*, counter the long-held idea that in hypertension "important vascular disease processes in women lag behind men by 10 to 20 years."[26] Their sex-specific analyses indicated that blood pressure measures actually progress more rapidly in women than in men, beginning early in life. And they suggest that this early onset difference between the sexes may contribute to later-life cardiovascular diseases that tend to present differently in women and men.

Additionally, researchers from Radboud University Medical Centre in the Netherlands found that in middle-aged women, hypertension symptoms are often mistaken for symptoms of menopause—leading to undertreatment of hypertension.[27]

According to another study, "Current guidelines do not suggest differential treatment of hypertension for women; however, a growing body of research suggests gender dimorphism in the pathophysiology of hypertension and pharmacological response to cardiovascular drugs. . . . [There are] frequently higher drug exposures in women and more frequent adverse drug reactions in all antihypertensive drug groups. As far as cardiovascular prevention is concerned, sex-specific data is often lacking in clinical trials."[28]

## RISKY OVERSIGHTS IN STROKE TREATMENTS FOR WOMEN

One 2021 study, "Women with Large Vessel Occlusion Acute Ischemic Stroke Are Less Likely to Be Routed to Comprehensive Stroke Centers," found women don't get the same quality of care after a stroke as men do.[29] And a meta-analysis published in *JAMA Neurology* that same year, "Women in Stroke Trials—A Tale of Perpetual Inequity in Cardiovascular Research," lays out findings from examining sex disparities in 115 stroke trials published between 2010 and 2020. The conclusion: "Compelling evidence exists that researchers have underperformed in maintaining sex balance in cardiovascular research."[30]

## SCADS OF MISSED DIAGNOSES FOR SCAD

SCAD is a condition that affects younger to middle-aged women and is far more common in women than men. Historically, it's been overlooked as a cause of heart attack because it is relatively uncommon and often occurs in patients without atherosclerotic risk factors.

"If you were trained as a cardiologist more than 10 years ago, which still represents a lot of young people in practice, you were taught that this condition was extremely rare, mainly happened in women, mainly happened after a pregnancy, and basically you wouldn't see it," says Dr. Hayes in an interview on the Cardiovascular Research Foundation's website TCTMD.com, a comprehensive online resource on interventional cardiology.[31] "What's happened since then is a recognition that this is more common than we thought—we've just been missing it, angiographically and clinically—and it's a very important cause of heart attack among women under 50."

## TOO YOUNG, TOO HEALTHY?

In 2003, Katherine Leon survived a 90% blockage of her left main coronary artery caused by a spontaneous dissection just days after giving birth.[32] SCAD led to a heart attack and she had emergency double bypass surgery. But events did not unfold as promptly as that sentence may imply.

I had my second son in 2003 at age 38. About five weeks after giving birth I suddenly experienced classic heart attack symptoms. I went to the emergency room, where despite chest pains, arm numbness and breathing problems, the doctors said there was nothing wrong with me and sent me home. The tests they did weren't what was needed to find out what was wrong.

The symptoms persisted. A few days later I headed back to the ER—the pain was unbearable and it was hard to breathe. I was frightened. This time a female doctor paid attention. An explorative cardiac catheterization procedure revealed I had a blockage in a major artery; I was told I needed emergency heart bypass surgery.

I thought, "Are you kidding me? I may have tried one cigarette in my life. I didn't have cholesterol issues. I didn't have blood pressure issues. I am a runner."

The causes of SCAD are many—and not entirely understood. It appears there is a relationship to chronic migraine, and there may be a genetic component as well as a relationship to connective tissue and fibromuscular disorders. But there's no way to assess the risk for SCAD, and once it appears there is a persistent danger of another spontaneous tear sometime in the future.

These gaps in knowledge are being overcome. Until recently, there weren't enough identified cases (often a young woman's heart blockage or heart attack wasn't attributed to SCAD) to get a good understanding of the condition. That all changed when Leon decided to reach out on social media to other women who had survived heart attacks and to spread the word about SCAD to women everywhere. She was amazed to find other SCAD patients; a support group of women coalesced around Leon's initiative.

Then, six years after her bypass surgery, Leon attended a WomenHeart Science and Leadership Symposium at Mayo Clinic, where she met Dr. Hayes, who was committed to improving diagnosis and treatment of heart disease in women. Today, Dr. Hayes is an international expert on SCAD and lead researcher for the Mayo Clinic SCAD Research Program.

"I told Dr. Hayes that our SCAD group had 70 women with the condition and they were committed to participating in research," Leon said. "She was amazed, since the largest study done to date only had 43 participants. That sparked an innovative approach to gathering information on SCAD—using a virtual multicenter disease registry that worked with various social media networks to allow people with SCAD to share data on the disease."

"We never imagined there would be 1,000 female patients in our virtual registry," Dr. Hayes says. Today there are over 1,500.

Leon's initiative and Dr. Hayes's expertise have transformed SCAD from an unknown, undiagnosed disorder into something that is routinely taught in medical schools and cardiology training.

## SURGERY CUTS OUT WOMEN TOO

Whether the cause is SCAD or other cardiac problems, when treatment for heart disease demands open heart surgery, women are once again at a disadvantage. A study by researchers from Duke and the Johns Hopkins University School of Medicine looked at male and female patients from 2011 to 2019 who got a first-time coronary artery bypass graft.[33] They found that women were 14–22% less likely than men to undergo

grafting of the left internal mammary artery (LIMA) to the left ante-
rior descending (LAD) artery, complete revascularization, and multi-
arterial grafting—all associated with improved short- and/or long-term
outcomes. The discrepancy in care and outcomes is echoed by a 2023
study in *JAMA* that found that between 2011 and 2022, 23% of women
died or experienced complications after coronary artery bypass grafting
(CABG), also known as heart bypass surgery, compared with 17% of
men. Death during or soon after the operation, the primary outcome,
also was higher in women than in men—2.8% and 1.7%, respectively.

## CARELESS CARE

Lyn Behnke, the cardiovascular nurse practitioner we met earlier, has
had quite a cardio journey of her own. Here's her story.

> At 50 I had a triple bypass. It shocked me. Even though my job was
> working in primary care and critical care for years, I really didn't
> know my own cardiovascular risk profile; I didn't feel like it would
> happen to me.
>
> When it did, it took a while, but I recovered well and thought
> all was good. But one day, after a 10-mile bike, a three-mile walk,
> and picking dinner out of the garden, I started to feel nauseous and
> I had a funny feeling in my chest that wouldn't go away.
>
> I went to the nearest hospital in my little town and was diag-
> nosed as having a heart attack. They sent me to another facility for
> treatment and there a doctor performed an angioplasty that almost
> killed me. It happened because the doctor hadn't looked at my pre-
> vious scans and records or he would have realized the angioplasty
> shouldn't have been performed because of my medical history.
>
> I see women misdiagnosed all the time. I think everybody going

into a hospital system needs an advocate who can ask questions and say, "Hey, wait a minute, let's think about this."

## CARDIAC-RELATED MEDICINE MISTAKES

One example of what recent research has turned up: In a 2016 study in the American Heart Association's journal *Circulation Research*, Dr. Bairey Merz and colleagues found that women don't receive heart medications that dilate the blood vessels or lower heart rate as promptly as men do.[34] Administration of aspirin therapy, blood pressure medications (angiotensin-converting enzyme inhibitors, angiotensin receptor blockers, beta-blockers), diuretics (aldosterone inhibitors) and statins is frequently delayed. They also found evidence that indicates many drugs commonly used to treat cardiovascular disease in women, especially those that prevent blood clots and heart rhythm problems, are metabolized differently in women. That puts them at risk for increased negative side effects and may indicate that women need to have dosages adjusted. But doctors don't know much about what medicines are effective, what proper dosages are or what should be avoided.

As Dr. Wenger wrote in a 2020 editorial in *JAMA Cardiology*, "We must remember that the cardiovascular health of women involves more than sex-specific medical research. Research must also include the domains of a woman's beliefs and behaviors and their community features as well as economic, environmental, and ethical concerns and the legislative, political, public policy, and sociocultural forces that affect their lives. Women's equity . . . involves equity in research and prevention and equal access to care and treatments."[35]

Let's look at examples of other health conditions where women are under- or mistreated and hear from those who have had to battle to get care for themselves and care for patients.

## CHAPTER 7

# A Neurological Stew

## Sex Differences in the Brain, Pain, Migraine, Myalgic Encephalomyelitis/Chronic Fatigue Syndrome and Addiction

I have a brain and a uterus and I use both.

—*Patricia Schroeder, the first female*
*US representative elected from Colorado*

Although heart disease is the number one killer of women, it is not the only condition that is made more potentially disruptive—and even lethal—by the consistent lack of interest in and understanding of how various diseases appear in women and how best they should be treated.

This chapter explores how those differences influence the prevention, diagnosis and treatment of neurological diseases and conditions that are experienced by males and females, such as chronic pain, migraine, myalgic encephalomyelitis/chronic fatigue syndrome and addiction.

## THE BRAIN

The brain is a control center for emotions, cognition and expression of and reaction to outside stimuli, whether they're negative stressors or pleasures. It also reacts to internal messages and commands from the immune system, hormones and your cardiovascular and other organ systems. Social norms, cultural attitudes and gender-related expectations regarding behavior also influence the brain's expression of emotions and an individual's perception of what's going on in their own and other people's brains (and emotions).[1] There are a lot of variables.

But it wasn't until researchers like Larry Cahill, PhD, professor of neurobiology and behavior at UC Irvine, decided to do animal and human research on the function of the amygdalae, a pair of small almond-shaped regions deep in the brain that help regulate emotion and encode memories—especially intense emotional memories—that neurologists and other brain scientists began to seriously acknowledge the significant differences in the neural structures in men's and women's brains and the differences in function they cause. Dr. Cahill says:

> For the first half of my career I, like most neuroscientists, assumed that biological sex did not matter for understanding any brain processes outside those directly related to reproduction.
>
> It turns out that this assumption is completely false. Sex influences exist at all levels of mammalian brain function, including the human brain. So, my work for the past 20 years has focused on understanding sex influences in the specific domain of emotional memory, and in challenging all of research/medicine to start actively understanding, rather than denying, sex differences, especially since denying them disproportionately harms women.
>
> I discovered it mattered if you were a man or a woman when I was studying the amygdala. I was exploring neural mechanisms of memory formation for emotionally arousing events using neuropharmacological, neuropsychological, and brain imaging with PET scans and MRIs.
>
> Well, the scans showed that the stress response is not the same in men and women. I noticed something funny when I showed men and women the same emotional stuff and scanned them. Activity in the amygdala in the right hemisphere was better at predicting if men would remember what they saw and it was the opposite for women.
>
> I started looking at all the literature available, and, wow, I saw that there are actually sex influences everywhere in neuroscience, except we don't know it or believe it. Furthermore, we in the field are overwhelmingly studying the male in animal studies and implying the results apply to men and women.

What open-minded brain scientists like Dr. Cahill have found shows that there are profound differences in men's and women's brains that influence everything from mental health (women are more prone to depression, men to autism spectrum disorder) to the ability to recognize faces (women are better at it than men, especially with other women).[2] But perhaps no brain-related health issue has been more dramatically affected by gender stereotypes and the lack of good science than the neurology of pain.

## DEFICIENT PAIN CARE

Women with acute and chronic pain often find their complaints are trivialized or dismissed—and if they are heard, it takes longer to get doctors to pay attention and to offer treatment. A 2008 study that looked at nearly 1,000 ER patient records found that women who complained of acute abdominal pain were given powerful opioid pain relievers 25% less often than men with similar complaints.[3]

In 2013, researchers from the University of Florida Pain Research and Intervention Center of Excellence looked at available research on sex and pain and found that both clinical studies and epidemiological work revealed that women have a greater risk for chronic pain and may in fact experience pain more severely.[4] They also stated that there was evidence of differences between men and women in response to pain treatments. But while the researchers concluded that biopsychosocial mechanisms, including sex hormones, endogenous opioid function, genetic factors, pain coping and catastrophizing (it seems they had to sneak that hysterical woman label back in there) and gender roles contribute to these sex differences in pain, they stated: "At present, the available evidence does not support sex-specific tailoring of treatments; however, this is a conceivable outcome in the foreseeable future."

Add to that the extra disregard that women of color and other marginalized groups face, and, as Jennifer Tsai—yet again in a wise article in *Scientific American*—explained in 2018: "Black patients really are getting less pain medication, and yes, *because* of their race. But this has nothing to do with genetic susceptibility. Such racial logic fuels stereotypes that feed inequity."[5]

Backing her up, a study in *Annals of Emergency Medicine* found that while 74% of white patients with a long bone fracture received pain relievers, only 57% of Black patients did, despite similar pain complaints noted in their medical records. Furthermore, the risk of receiving no pain relief at all while in the emergency department was 66% greater for Black patients than for white patients.[6]

Members of the LGBTQ community also face discrimination when it comes to treating their pain. It stems from a combination of ignorance, lack of training and bias against nonconforming gender orientation. A 2018 survey of medical school students found that 80% of them felt either "not competent" or only "somewhat competent" to provide care to patients with non-cis gender or sex issues.[7]

Practicing doctors have no better interaction with or understanding of health issues facing the LGBTQ community. One study found that only 5% of doctors asked patients about their sexual history; only around a third of doctors could say if they had lesbian patients, and just over 10% said they knew anything about lesbian-specific health issues.[8]

## PAIN AND TRANS MEDICAL CARE

In a 2019 article, updated in 2021, "How to Provide Effective Pain Management to LGBTQ Individuals," Danielle Weitzer, DO, with a residency in psychiatry, shared her personal and clinical experience.

Throughout medical school and the years following, I underwent several surgical procedures, some of which helped me to physically transition from male to female and others to correct complications from those surgeries. During this time, I continued to face discrimination in medical school as many classmates did not understand my overall transition.

I grew afraid to see medical providers for my growing number of problems. I was too fearful of more rejection or discrimination. Complications from my surgeries have ranged from getting burned to neck pain and nose pain, including having difficulty breathing. My nose was and continues to be painful anytime I sneeze or attempt to blow. In addition, I developed sharp pain for many months, especially pronounced while dilating my new genitals.

To this day, I continue to struggle with pain and embarrassment of these areas.[9]

Her medical and psychiatric training has fueled her determination to increase awareness of the lack of research on chronic pain in the LGBTQ community. She's committed to making the medical profession aware that transgender individuals are at more risk for pain conditions than the general population. Plus, because they often have multiple surgeries, postoperative pain is an issue. There are also greater risks for mental health issues—which often correlate with increased pain syndromes—in patients who transition.

### HEALTHYWOMEN TACKLES PAIN

In July 2019 at the HealthyWomen Chronic Pain Summit,[10] Kaveeta Vasisht, MD, PharmD, acting associate commissioner of the FDA's Office of Women's Health, stated, "The pain community at large is still in the early stages of female-centered research. Even within the FDA's Office of Women's Health, established in 1994, only 31% of its research projects have looked at sex differences to date."[11]

In that symposium, HealthyWomen presented a survey of more than 1,000 women living with chronic pain. It found that while 90% had received a diagnosis for the cause of their pain:

- 36% of respondents said they do not think their healthcare provider takes their pain seriously, while 45% believe their provider is "somewhat understanding" and 17% say their HCP is *not* understanding.
- 62% reported they sometimes feel hopeless and/or helpless about their pain, while 35% said they always feel hopeless and/or helpless.
- 38% said that they do not have access to enough information about pain.

When asked what changes in pain care are important to them, they said they would like to see:

- adequately trained providers (65%)
- support from their healthcare provider (58%)
- increased availability of resources (56%).

"As a practicing healthcare professional, I am not surprised to learn that women place 'adequately trained providers' at the top of their list when it comes to pain management," said HealthyWomen CEO Beth Battaglino, RN-C. "There is always more to learn, especially when it comes to chronic pain that's not linked to something visible or related to a diagnosis like cancer."

A small 2021 study (mostly middle-aged white participants), titled "Gender Biases in Estimation of Others' Pain," revealed that when male and female patients express the same amount of pain, in the general population both males and females say that the females' pain is less intense and more likely to benefit from psychotherapy versus medication as compared to men's pain.[12]

One of that study's authors, Elizabeth A. Reynolds Losin, PhD, from the Department of Psychology at the University of Miami, explained it this way: "If the stereotype is to think women are more expressive than men, perhaps 'overly' expressive, then the tendency will be to discount women's pain behaviors. The flip side of this stereotype is that men are perceived to be stoic, so when a man makes an intense pain facial expression, you think, 'Oh my, he must be dying!'"[13]

That disparity in response to men and women's pain may contribute to the findings of a 2022 study titled "Sex and Race Differences in the Evaluation and Treatment of Young Adults Presenting to the Emergency Department with Chest Pain." It found that on average when a woman shows up to an ER complaining of chest pain, she has to wait 29% longer than a man with similar symptoms to be evaluated for a possible heart attack.

## "THE GIRL WHO CRIED PAIN"—ONE MORE TIME

In 2001, Diane E. Hoffmann, JD MS, Jacob A. France Professor of Health Care Law and director of the Law & Health Care Program at the University of Maryland, was a co-author with bioethicist Anita Tarzian, PhD, RN, of an article titled "The Girl Who Cried Pain: A Bias Against Women in the Treatment of Pain," published in the *Journal of Law, Medicine & Ethics*.[14] It explored the possibility that there were quantifiable differences in the biological and psychosocial origins of pain in men and women. Looking at available literature, they found that women were more likely than men to report migraine and chronic tension headaches, facial pain, musculoskeletal pain and pain from osteoarthritis, rheumatoid arthritis and fibromyalgia. They also saw that in clinical trials women had lower pain thresholds and lower pain tolerance than men.

Do women report such aches and pains more because they experience them more or because they are more willing to say they are in pain? That's a bit of a toss-up, says Hoffmann.

"We started looking at what scientists knew that could explain the differences in men's and women's pain experience and that got broadened to cultural and social differences," says Hoffmann. "That included differences in reporting pain and in how pain is talked about.

"It became clear that given that women have more severe pain and their chronic pain is often different than men's, they should be treated better," she adds. "But there's a paradox: Pain is more of a problem for women, yet they receive less treatment for it. It should be the other way around."

In 2022, Hoffmann and co-authors Roger Fillingim, PhD, professor and director of the Pain Research and Intervention Center of Excellence at the University of Florida, and Christin Veasley, co-founder and director of the Chronic Pain Research Alliance, dove back in and looked at the progress made in understanding the sex and gender influences on pain and pain management. Their article was titled "The Woman Who Cried Pain: Do Sex-Based Disparities Still Exist in the Experience and Treatment of Pain?"[15]

"We looked at what we learned in the past 20 years," says Hoffmann. "For example, we know women have more pain of longer duration. So one area we looked at was research into the biological pathways that affect pain. We discovered research showing that sex hormones have complex effects on pain-related responses and that there are sex differences in mechanisms whereby immune function, genes, neurochemical processes and brain structure and function mediate pain pathways."

The article tackled five points:

1. It looked at what has been learned in the past 20 years regarding pain and the pain experience.
2. It explored what studies have found about the biological and psychosocial differences between men and women that relate to the experience of pain.
3. They examined the available literature on gender- and sex-based disparities in pain treatment and what that literature reveals about how much of a problem it still is.
4. They also explored explanations for why healthcare providers treat pain in men differently from pain in women.
5. Then they made recommendations on how to improve the treatment of pain in women and lessen sex-based disparities.

"Overall, the more we learn about pain the more complex it is," says Hoffmann. "We found some progress had been made, but much is still not understood about the biological and psychosocial underpinnings of differences in the pain experience and pain reporting between men and women." The 2022 article concluded:

• Some studies in the past two decades do indicate important disparities in pain treatment and in the studies available none found that men were ever treated less well for pain than women.

- Solid studies are available that show implicit bias at work in response to women in pain on the part of medical students and residents.

The bottom line: "More research and education are needed before pain treatment for women and men improves," says Hoffmann. "When doctors can't explain what is happening they are more likely to say it is all in your head or that it's no big deal. All people deserve high-quality, effective pain treatment, but women, in particular, seem to have more difficulty obtaining such care."

Dismissing pain complaints as an emotional reaction or "hysteria" means that cardiovascular problems, headaches, migraine, chronic pain from hard-to-detect causes, such as fibromyalgia and myalgic encephalomyelitis/chronic fatigue syndrome (ME/CFS), musculoskeletal pain and gynecological issues, are often overlooked or misdiagnosed.

### PRECISION PAIN MANAGEMENT: INNOVATION THAT MAY REMOVE BIAS

By now, hundreds of studies have shown that men and women—in fact all people with chronic pain—have physiological differences in the way their brain and spinal cord process sensory information, and that, says Veasley, "is one of the most transformative research findings this field has ever had." Veasley continued:

> We can now definitively state those with chronic pain—regardless of whether an initiating event or underlying cause can be pinpointed—are experiencing a "real" medical condition.
>
> Chronic pain is not due to weakness or a psychological issue, although we do know that a person's psyche influences the severity

and trajectory of chronic pain, just like it does in all chronic illnesses. We now have scientific evidence that people who develop chronic pain have neurological systems that do not function in the same way as those who don't experience chronic pain, including altered influences from the immune and endocrine systems.

This line of research has helped to legitimize the biological basis of chronic pain as a disease in its own right—and finally, people are not dismissing chronic pain as "all in one's head," even if altered neurological patterns may originate in the brain.

## REDEFINING PAIN

This deeper understanding of pain's origins and manifestation has led to acceptance of newer concepts of pain.[16] These new concepts are central sensitization, persistent acute pain, nociplastic pain and chronic overlapping pain conditions—and they all seem to affect women more than men.

- **Central sensitization** causes pain to be experienced with widespread, heightened sensitivity and with less ability of the body's inhibitory pathways to dampen or suppress pain perception. It turns out that the peripheral nervous system has limited input in central sensitization, but the central nervous system reacts as if there has been an intense or high level of pain stimulation. Recent studies show that this also amplifies the neural signaling so that a person becomes hypersensitive.[17] Even the most gentle touch can cause pain.
- **Persistent acute pain** can trigger amplified neural signaling, but it can also arise from less identifiable causes. While spinal cord injury and stroke have long been known to

be possible triggers, it is now clear that conditions that mostly or exclusively affect women, such as migraine and chronic tension headaches, endometriosis and rheumatoid arthritis, as well as fibromyalgia, irritable bowel syndrome and chronic fatigue syndrome, seem to be associated with central sensitization as well.[18] As Hoffmann points out in her 2022 follow-up study, "Central sensitization highlights the limitations of prior conceptualizations of pain, which viewed pain primarily as a symptom of actual or potential tissue damage."

- **Nociplastic pain** is pain that "arises from altered [pain sensation] despite no clear evidence of actual or threatened tissue damage . . . or evidence for disease or lesion . . . causing the pain." This is a new definition, introduced in 2020 by the International Association for the Study of Pain (IASP), clearly establishing that nociplastic pain is a newly recognized subtype of pain.[19] IASP identifies fibromyalgia, complex regional pain syndrome, nonspecific chronic low-back pain, temporomandibular disorders, and irritable bowel syndrome as frequent causes of nociplastic pain and body-wide hypersensitivity.

- **Chronic overlapping pain conditions** (COPCs) are another area where there's been progress in understanding pain. Research shows that if a woman has one pain condition, she is more likely to develop a second or third. Frequent COPCs include vulvodynia, temporomandibular disorders, myalgic encephalomyelitis/chronic fatigue syndrome, irritable bowel syndrome, interstitial cystitis/painful bladder syndrome, fibromyalgia, endometriosis, chronic tension-type headache, chronic migraine headache and chronic low back pain.[20]

In 2020, for the first time since 1979, IASP issued a revised definition of pain: "An unpleasant sensory and emotional experience associated with, or resembling that associated with, actual or potential tissue damage," and it added six key notes to further clarify the definition[21]:

- Pain is always a personal experience that is influenced to varying degrees by biological, psychological and social factors.
- Pain and nociception are different phenomena. Pain cannot be inferred solely from activity in sensory neurons.
- Through their life experiences, individuals learn the concept of pain.
- A person's report of an experience of pain should be respected.
- Although pain usually serves an adaptive role, it may have adverse effects on function and social and psychological well-being.
- Verbal description is only one of several behaviors to express pain; inability to communicate does not negate the possibility that a human or a nonhuman animal experiences pain.

## OBJECTIVE TESTING

The next step to remove bias from evaluation of pain syndromes is already underway at Indiana University.[22] Researchers there are working on developing an objective way to assess blood biomarkers that indicate pain severity so that anyone can receive precision pain management. The good news is that some of the biomarkers for pain are targets of already existing drugs, such as a tricyclic antidepressant and supplements such as B6, B12 and a plant flavonoid.

## OTHER NEUROLOGICAL CONDITIONS: MIGRAINE, MYALGIC ENCEPHALOMYELITIS/CHRONIC FATIGUE SYNDROME (ME/CFS) AND ADDICTION

While pain is a component of migraine, ME/CFS and addiction, they each have distinct attributes as well—and each condition has been ignored, dismissed or misdiagnosed in women over and over again.

### *Migraine*

Migraine syndrome (researchers now realize it is far more than just a headache) is characterized by nerve-controlled inflammation of the dura, the membrane between the brain and the skull. Seventy percent of migraine sufferers are women, and they pay a price. According to a 2018 report from SWHR, migraine headaches cost the United States an estimated $78 billion annually, with women accounting for about 80% of direct medical and lost labor costs.[23]

A genetic predisposition is often present and a study using brain MRIs supports the idea that male and female brains are differentially affected by migraine, and the differences involve both brain structure and functional circuits.[24]

A headache is a well-documented migraine symptom, but not everyone who has a migraine gets a headache. Migraine can also involve visual disturbances; nausea and vomiting; dizziness; sensitivity to light, noise and smell; and temporary weakness on one side. About 25% of people with migraine experience an aura, or visual disturbances. For women under age 50, migraine with aura increases the risk of stroke, especially if they smoke or use oral contraceptives.

Hormones play a major role as triggers. For example, a dip in estrogen levels before menstruation is associated with onset of migraine. A 2021 study presented at the 7th Congress of the European Academy of Neurology found that pregnant women with migraine are at higher risk of obstetric and postnatal complications.[25]

A 2023 study in *Neurology* sheds some light on what may be happening: fluctuations in estrogen levels around menstruation may increase levels of a protein that widens blood vessels in the brain, one of the series of physiological changes that lead to migraine.[26] But that isn't the whole story.

Martha Nolan, senior policy advisor at HealthyWomen who served as vice president of public policy at SWHR, says there is still much to learn about hormones' impact on migraine: "For some women, the fluctuation of estrogen levels around menstruation and menopause can trigger a migraine attack. For others, it can dampen the intensity. Because estrogen is responsible for controlling pain sensation, it has been shown that taking certain types of birth control and also menopause can help ameliorate the severity of a migraine attack. Yet for some women, the exact opposite happens. Researchers are working hard to try to figure the fluctuation connection out—but they don't have answers yet."[27]

## SILENT SUFFERING

Lindsay Weitzel, PhD, is the founder of MigraineNation and the MigraineNation Patient Navigator Program and a migraine sufferer who experienced her first migraine at age four. As she recalled:

> My first memory of a migraine is from around the age of four and it just hit me. I lived in a small town and although my family did take me to a lot of specialists, they each just thought about their specialty. One neurologist thought I was just making it up and I have a specific memory of [a] pediatrician telling me, "You are

perfectly happy!" Another pediatrician once said—right in front of me—"Sometimes these kids that complain a lot when nothing is wrong have lupus." What? Nothing wrong? Lupus?

The experience of constant migraine caused me to develop complex regional pain syndrome (a ceaseless pain like burning fire) down the right side of my face, head, neck and arm. The doctors didn't see that either—and the combination was terrible.

But by the time I was in third grade I knew that I didn't want to be called a hypochondriac, so I stopped speaking about my headaches and the burning sensation until I was 17. No one knew how much pain I was in.

Then at 17 I was given an Imitrex injection and it worked for the migraine but not for the burning pain sensation. Eventually I had multiple rhizotomies that killed the nerve fibers responsible for sending those burning pain signals to my brain. My face and eye stopped burning, the migraines lessened—I was taking Topamax— and now the migraines are episodic, not constant.

I tell people you have to go back over and over to find the right combo of treatments that work for you. And you have to find the right way for you to express what you are experiencing so that the doctors understand.

Once again, the burden of proof rests on the female patient's shoulders.

Disparities in the diagnosis of migraine and in patient care are centered around gaps in information about sex, gender, race and ethnicity.[28] In 2018, to address the missing information, Monica Mallampalli, PhD, who served as the vice president of scientific affairs at the Society for Women's Health Research (SWHR) before serving as chair of HealthyWomen's chronic pain advisory council, held a Science,

Technology and Innovation Roundtable in Baltimore, Maryland, to discuss migraine therapies in women.[29]

"Sex differences haves been studied in migraine to some extent, but there is a need for more basic researchers to focus on [the] pathophysiology of migraine disease," says Dr. Mallampalli. "Migraines could be hormonal for men too—we don't know. And while there are some new medications, they don't work for everyone. HealthyWomen is focused on exploring noninvasive nondrug treatments for women and there's just a lot more we need to understand."

## MYALGIC ENCEPHALOMYELITIS/CHRONIC FATIGUE SYNDROME

When it comes to missed diagnoses and misdiagnoses, myalgic encephalomyelitis, also known as chronic fatigue syndrome and commonly referred to as ME/CFS, is another solid example of how systemic prejudices and lack of rigorous science harm women and diminish healthcare. ME/CFS is a chronic neurological condition that affects both the nervous and immune systems. According to the Department of Health and Human Services' Office on Women's Health, women are two to four times more likely than men to be diagnosed with ME/CFS—and there are no Food and Drug Administration (FDA)—approved treatments specifically for treating ME/CFS. What exists simply tries to address symptoms, not the underlying cause(s).

Art Mirin, PhD, a former computational scientist at Lawrence Livermore National Laboratory, points out that more times than not, many in the medical community have wrongly perceived the disease as being psychogenic.

This continues to happen even though in 2015 the Institute of Medicine (now the National Academy of Medicine) issued a comprehensive report characterizing ME/CFS as "a serious, chronic, complex, multisystem disease that frequently and dramatically limits the activities of affected patients."[30] They strongly refuted the dismissal that women with ME/CFS sometimes encounter in doctors' offices when describing their symptoms.

And, adds Dr. Mirin, we see the same mistake being made today in the analysis of women who complain of long COVID syndrome. "Unfortunately, women continue to be treated poorly compared to men," says Dr. Mirin, "by being viewed as hysterical or having it all in their head."

## WHEN DOCTORS DON'T HAVE ANSWERS, PATIENTS DON'T GET TREATMENT

For decades Rivka Solomon has had to contend with the challenges of obtaining a diagnosis for and treatment of ME/CFS.

When I was 21, two of my college roommates and I got mononucleosis at the same time. They got better in a couple of months, and I never got better. I'm 60 now.

For a full year I could barely stand up and no one was sure why. It was diagnosed as chronic mono, then chronic Epstein-Barr virus, then chronic fatigue syndrome. And now they call it ME/CFS, myalgic encephalomyelitis/chronic fatigue syndrome. Most of us just call it ME. But whatever you call it, there are as many as 2.5 million people in the United States with ME, and 75 percent of them are women.

We have no treatments, no cure, and people can be sick and disabled for decades, often bedridden like me, some unable to care for or feed themselves. That first year when I developed the post-infection chronic illness I went to a doctor who had no experience with what I was presenting; I was her first ME patient. So she was willing to try some out-of-the-box things, Chinese medicines, etc. Nothing helped. But after about a year I spontaneously got well enough to get out of bed—no one knows why, but that does happen sometimes.

I then experienced seven years of semi-remission. It was not a full remission, as I was still dragging myself around, exhausted all the time, but I would work, play, travel, even though I was often wiped out. Every now and then I would spend a few days bedridden and didn't know why.

Then in the winter of 1990, when I was in grad school, I got a cold. The cold turned into bronchitis and that turned into walking pneumonia, relaunching full ME all over again. I have never gotten over that.

I spent the next two years in and out of bed and was so weak I couldn't carry my own books to class. After graduating, and for the last three decades, I have been so sick that I have been in or near bed much of the time.

Today, there are still no FDA-approved treatments. That's what happens when the government refuses to take an illness seriously. And that attitude infiltrates everywhere. Only a third of medical schools teach about infection-associated chronic illness, such as ME/CFS and now long COVID, and still many or most doctors wrongly think ME is a psychological illness. It's not!

What role does sexism play in this? I don't have the answer. But if men are deciding which illnesses to fund, perhaps they tend to be those that affect men, and other health conditions that they don't understand can more easily get dismissed as "all in your head."

The medical profession's confrontation with long COVID may be changing that. Up to one in eight people who contract COVID-19 develop long COVID, a post-viral infection syndrome that causes persistent fatigue and cognition problems—just like ME/CFS does.[31] And finally, as Akiko Iwasaki, PhD, the Sterling Professor of Immunobiology at the Yale School of Medicine, said, "The pandemic has opened the world's eye to the fact that many chronic illnesses have been largely ignored, dismissed, and ridiculed. Long COVID has taught the world that these diseases are real, there is a biological basis for them, and we need to study them."[32]

No healthcare organization is leading the way more than Mayo Clinic. Recently, #MEAction and Mayo Clinic applied for a grant from the Society to Improve Diagnosis in Medicine to transform the diagnostic and treatment process for people with ME/CFS.[33] The grant allowed a diagnostic and treatment algorithm to be built that provides physicians with an interactive flowchart that presents optimal steps in diagnosing and treating patients, especially those with severe symptoms of the condition.

## ADDICTION

There are three stages of addiction progression—binge/intoxication, withdrawal/negative affect and preoccupation/anticipation—and sex differences are evident in all of them, according to both animal and human studies. Clinical studies show women become dependent on opioids and alcohol more quickly than men, most likely because of differences in metabolism as well as in how drugs are absorbed and eliminated. That could all be a result of differences in body fat to water ratios in men and women, women's smaller body size and sex differences in the brain's electric and chemical circuitry that regulate the ability to feel pleasure and reward. Hormones are also a factor: research shows that ovarian hormones, such as estradiol, interact with nicotinic receptors, and that changes how they function.[34]

There are also sex differences in the response to certain addictive drugs. One study that used brain scans to track how smoking affects the pleasure-producing neurotransmitter dopamine in men and women's brains found that nicotine impacts dopamine in men's and women's brains at different rates and in different locations.[35] Women's response happens in the area of the brain associated with habit formation, while men's happens in an area that heightens the effects of nicotine. The National Institute of Drug Abuse (NIDA) says that women have a harder time quitting smoking than men do, likely because they metabolize nicotine faster than men. That's also a possible explanation for why nicotine replacement patches and gums work better in men than women.[36]

Societal norms and pressures shape differences in women's and men's addiction experiences too—impacting substance abuse, relapse and treatment seeking. For example, because more women are primary caregivers, it makes those with addiction issues less likely to be able to reach out for help and complete addiction treatment that would take them away from their duties at home. Another factor fueling women's struggles with addiction is physical abuse at the hands of their partner. A third of women experience such trauma, and it is known to fuel obesity, chronic pain, depression and substance use.[37] Research also indicates that differences in response to addiction treatment for trans women comes from life circumstances. And for all women, when stressors are recognized treatment is more effective.[38]

Providing treatment for addiction also needs to take into account sex and gender differences in biochemistry. When it comes to getting off drugs, some studies show that sex differences in the production of stress hormones such as cortisol make women's experience of withdrawal harsher and fuel stress-induced relapses, which are more frequent in women than men.

Whatever the cause, NIDA concludes that when women do enter treatment for addiction, they are generally experiencing more severe medical, behavioral, psychological and social problems. NIDA suggests that's because they progress more rapidly from first use of an addictive substance to dependence or addiction.[39]

The bottom line, so artfully expressed in the conclusion of the executive summary of a 2019 FDA meeting, Opioid and Nicotine Use, Dependence, and Recovery: Influences of Sex and Gender: "Finally, and perhaps most importantly, data gaps still exist in our knowledge of the impact of sex and gender on substance use and misuse. There is a dearth of information on the basic neurobiology of the impact of sex differences in animal models of opioid and nicotine use. Although there is a wealth of research on nicotine and opioid use and recovery in humans, there is inconsistent reporting and analysis by gender. We do not know if sex and gender differences exist in many areas of research simply because many researchers may not be aware of the ubiquitous influences of sex and gender and have not performed the relevant statistical analyses to detect those differences."[40]

# CHAPTER 8

Depression and Anxiety

## The Physical and Social Determinants of Women's Mental Health

It's my experience that people are a lot more sympathetic
if they can see you hurting, and for the millionth time in
my life I wish for measles or smallpox or some other easily
understood disease just to make it easier on me and also on
them.

> —*A teenager contending with bipolar disorder in
> Jennifer Niven's novel* All the Bright Places[1]

D epression and its cousin anxiety are far more common in women than men. It's estimated that in the United States, women (10.4%) are nearly twice as likely as men (5.5%) to contend with depression in any year, and when it comes to a major depressive episode, women are again far more likely to be afflicted.[2]

That's true of anxiety as well: Women may be two to three times more likely to experience generalized anxiety disorder (GAD) and panic disorder than men, they meet lifetime criteria for social anxiety disorder (SAD) more than men, and they have more severe symptoms of all forms of anxiety.[3]

Yet we are just beginning to understand the mix of genetics, metabolic systems, the gut biome, inflammation, hormones and environmental and cultural forces that create sex differences in frequency and manifestation of depression and anxiety. It has taken years to stop attributing women's health issues to hysteria—a hugely misogynistic and misplaced mental health diagnosis—and begin to pay respectful and medically accurate attention to mental health issues such as depression and anxiety.

## WOMEN'S UNIQUE MENTAL HEALTH DYNAMICS

To understand why women are more likely to experience depression than men, a good place to start is the six Ps: puberty, premenstrual cycles, pregnancy, postpartum depression, perimenopause and postmenopause.

Whenever a woman experiences shifts in sex hormones—as happens in puberty, with the monthly menstrual cycle, during pregnancy, during postpartum, and before and after menopause—there are changes in neurotransmitters (which influence mood) and neurosteroids.[4] Neurosteroids affect how neurons fire in the brain, and they're thought to play a role in the development of major depression, post-traumatic stress disorder, premenstrual dysphoric disorder (PMDD) and postpartum depression.

Sex hormones also play a role in anxiety. Changing levels of progesterone and estrogen during the menstrual cycle and over a lifetime can influence the development—and severity—of anxiety disorders.[5] Pregnancy is associated with an increased risk for GAD, and if a woman had either GAD or SAD before becoming pregnant, she is at an increased risk for postpartum depression and anxiety disorders.[6] It may be that in some women, such shifts in hormone levels—both up and down—are triggered by genetic dysregulation, which increases their susceptibility to depression and anxiety.

A 2017 study by researchers from the National Institute of Mental Health's behavioral endocrinology branch that came out in *Molecular Psychiatry* found that to be the case. It showed that dysregulation of certain genes was the root cause of PMDD. "This is a big moment for women's health, because it establishes that women with PMDD have an intrinsic difference in their molecular apparatus for response to sex hormones—not just emotional behaviors they should be able to voluntarily control," declared one of the researchers, David Goldman, MD.[7]

This is joined by a study in the spring of 2023 that revealed genetic differences in men's and women's risk for depression. Researchers from McGill University looked at more than 270,000 people and discovered that while males have one area of DNA linked to depression, females have 11.[8] Furthermore, it turns out that depression has a direct connection to the development of metabolic diseases in women. That insight may lead to new ways of treating women with depression.

## BEYOND BIOLOGY

Environmental pressures are also important triggers. In our society, factors that make women more vulnerable to depression and anxiety include body shaming, being the target of violence, childhood sexual abuse and overall lack of gender equality. Adding to that, the COVID-19 pandemic and current social upheavals appear to have led to high rates of emotional turmoil. From January 4 to 16, 2023, around 31% of US women reported symptoms of an anxiety disorder, only 10 points lower than the peak week in October 2020, when 41.8% said they had such symptoms.[9]

Other factors that influence the development of depression and anxiety involve women's experience and response to the many stressors they face socially and economically. And those factors are compounded when a woman is a member of a marginalized ethnic or racial community.

According to the Department of Health and Human Services' Office on Women's Health, "Women are more likely than men to report symptoms of stress, including headaches and upset stomach. Women are also more likely to have mental health conditions that are made worse by stress, such as depression or anxiety."[10]

MRIs show that women have a stronger stress response in the limbic/striatal regions of the brain while men have a stronger stress response in their prefrontal cortex. As a result, there are different brain processes going on, and that indicates that different approaches to treatment might be appropriate. Not that anyone knows exactly what those might be.

## GAPS IN TREATMENT

Lack of knowledge about the underlying causes of depression and anxiety in women is not the only gap in the appropriate diagnosis and treatment of women. There is also an astounding lack of information on appropriate medications and optimal dosages of antidepression and anti-anxiety medications.

While we know women are more than twice as likely as men to use antidepressants, according to an analysis from the National Center for Health Statistics, there are no antidepressant or anti-anxiety medications made specifically to treat these conditions in women. In addition, there are not dose-for-sex recommendations for available medications, and the only specific risks or needs that are addressed are those relating to warnings about taking some medications during pregnancy or while breastfeeding.

We do know a little bit about the different effects antidepression medications have on women and men. For example, there are studies that show women respond better to SSRIs such as Zoloft than men do, but men are more responsive to tricyclics like Elavil.[11]

Furthermore, we know that women have less stomach acid than men, so when they take antidepressants, the drug can be more quickly absorbed into their body—increasing the risk for toxicity. The fact that women in general carry more body fat may also affect how antidepressants are metabolized—the body fat can hold the medications in the body for a longer period of time.[12] But that's about it.

Clearly, the medical and research communities need to look into the sex-related pharmacology of medications as well as sex and gender differences in vulnerability to depression and anxiety.

## DEPRESSION'S LINK TO HEART DISEASE

Depression and anxiety carry an increased risk of cardiovascular disease, and when a woman who is depressed or anxious experiences a cardiac event, the outcome is more adverse for her than for a male counterpart—especially if she is a younger woman.[13] Conversely, after having a heart attack or stroke, more women than men experience depression.

Clearly, mental and physical health are intertwined, and to be able to fully optimize women's well-being, the interplay must be considered in research and clinical treatment.

## CODA: FINDING RELIEF

Although therapy and medication are often essential and lifesaving components of treatment for chronic depression and anxiety, there are also self-help tools at hand.

Jeremy Nobel, MD, PhD, a faculty member of the Harvard School of Public Health and the Harvard Medical School, is founder and president of the Foundation for Art and Healing.[1] The foundation's signature initiative, the UnLonely Project, addresses the personal and public health challenges of loneliness and social isolation, conditions that are intertwined with depression and anxiety, by helping people leverage the relationship between creative expression and health and well-being.

My story reinforces the power of creativity to help women manage depression and anxiety. For me the way to manage my mental health was (and is) through painting. I knew my husband, Bob, had Alzheimer's disease before anyone else did, including Bob. He was only 65 years old, but he had some of the telltale symptoms, including forgetfulness and absentmindedness, which were highly unusual for him. But when Bob went to see a neurologist, he was told everything was fine, that his symptoms were just a normal part of aging. I knew the neurologist was wrong.

Around this time, I happened to be putting on a women's health panel featuring a physician who was an expert on Alzheimer's. I set up an appointment for Bob with this doctor, and we quickly had the dreaded but accurate diagnosis: Alzheimer's disease.

For a few years after the diagnosis, Bob was OK. Not great, but well enough to travel with me and live a somewhat normal life, although not independently—I was always by his side. But he deteriorated, as one with Alzheimer's always does, and eventually, it came time to move him into a memory care facility—a difficult decision if ever there was one, but one that I felt was best for Bob's health and general well-being. Bob stayed in the facility for a while, but I wasn't happy with his quality of life there. Ultimately, I decided that he would be best off at home, with me and a train of round-the-clock caregivers.

It may have been my husband's body in the house with me, but the man in the house was not my husband. This man was but a hollowed out, cracked shell of my husband. He didn't even really look like Bob. The strapping smile, the confident posture, the ability to be effortlessly laid back—all deleted like some old copy in one of his stories that never made it to press.

Though I was never alone, and I had plenty to occupy myself between work and my social life, there was a loneliness to my days and a gnawing guilt combined with a kind of grief in reverse. Bob was still alive, but I missed him, and I also at times resented the helpless, crazed person he'd become. And then I felt bad about that because, of course, he was an innocent victim in all of this.

One thing helped buoy me. I've always loved to paint and found myself profoundly drawn to the canvas during Bob's decline. Painting blocked out the rest of the world and provided me with a launchpad for the mornings. Often when I'd wake up, the first thing on my mind was how I'd continue the painting I left off the day before.

While Bob was dying (because really, that's what was happening during all those 15 brutal years that he was slipping away), I spent much of my free time absorbed in making art. Since Bob passed in March 2022, I've continued painting and have even sold some of my work.

Right now, I'm in a bit of a rut with painting and with my grief. Work is good. Friends are good. I have this book coming out and other exciting things on the horizon. But I don't know what to do with one particular half-done painting. I don't like it as it is, and I know I need to change it, but I don't know what to do with it. One of these days, I'll throw black paint over it and start over. That's the thing about me. I never leave things unfinished. And if I don't like something, I always fix it so that I do. It's just a matter of getting to the place where I can start again. It has to come to me. I know it will. And painting will carry me there.

# CHAPTER 9

# Women's Uniqueness

## Fibroids, Endometriosis, Pregnancy and Postmenopause

What sets you apart can sometimes feel like a burden and, it's not. A lot of the time, it's what makes you great.

—*Emma Stone*

Dr. Nanette Wenger, professor emerita at Emory University School of Medicine, consultant at the Emory Heart and Vascular Center and founding consultant at Emory Women's Heart Center and SWHR, led the fight against "bikini medicine," but equally concerning was the lack of sex-specific research into conditions that exclusively or disproportionately affect women.

This lack of information persists on how fibroids develop and how to best treat them, how pregnancy interacts with the neurobiology and endocrinology of women, how various medications affect the fetus and the mother and how everything from puberty to menopause affects brain health and the immune system.

In this chapter, I have chosen to write about fibroids, endometriosis, pregnancy and postmenopause. These four health issues collectively affect most women.

- Almost 80% of women will develop fibroids sometime during their childbearing years.[1]
- Endometriosis, which happens when tissue similar to the lining of the uterus grows outside the uterus, may affect over 11% of American women between ages 15 and 44, according to the Department of Health and Human Services' Office on Women's Health.[2]
- The Centers for Disease Control and Prevention says that in 2022 there were around 6,370,000 pregnancies in the United States, with 4,131,000 live births, 1,152,000 induced

abortions and 1,087,000 fetal losses.[3] And the number of live births, maternal deaths and pregnancy-related complications is on the rise, post-*Roe*.[4]

• And 85% of all women report experiencing some menopause-related symptoms.[5]

For any one woman to truly thrive, all women must thrive, and—why is this not more obvious to folks—for men to thrive, both men and women must be treated well and wisely.

## FIGURING OUT FIBROIDS

Between 70% and 80% of women will develop fibroids by age 50. While many fibroids are asymptomatic, they can cause life-altering pain, interfere with fertility and cause physical and emotional problems. But no one knows exactly why these benign tumors appear, how to catch them early to prevent their overgrowth or how to guarantee that removing them won't interfere with a woman's fertility or well-being.

"There are so many variables to consider—from the size and location of the fibroids, to a patient's age, a woman's goals and her desire to give birth in the future," explains Soyini Hawkins, MD, MPH, FACOG, founder of the Fibroid and Pelvic Wellness Center of Georgia. Unfortunately, those variables make getting prompt, effective treatment challenging.

## FROM PATIENT TO ADVOCATE

Shayla Defils, a fibroid patient and advocate for the fibroid awareness and advocacy organization the White Dress Project, is on doctor number four—and finally is getting the advice and care she needs.[6]

I was diagnosed in the Air Force reserves through a routine ultrasound. They said, "Oh, there are fibroids. Nothing to worry about. It will go away."

Then five years ago my periods had gotten so heavy that I went to a doctor to get an ablation done. Without really knowing anything she said, "We know cancer is common in Black women" and diagnosed me WITH CANCER.

I went immediately to get another opinion. That doctor did an ultrasound and the largest fibroid was the size of a SMALL grapefruit. Even though I was lethargic, and sometimes I couldn't leave the house, nothing was done. The doctor said, "Oh, you can live with it if it is not painful." She was not listening to me.

Because I found the White Dress Project I learned about alternatives to hysterectomies. And I realized that if the doctor isn't listening to you, make them hear you! Go armed with information and ask pointed questions. If that doesn't work, find another doctor.

The White Dress Project's founder and Peabody Award–winning journalist Tanika Gray Valbrun says, "I used to think the ignorance about and ignoring of the issues around fibroids was an old people thing—old doctors not being in this community and being quick to say, 'No, the pain isn't that bad,' or 'Calm down,' or 'Some women just bleed like that.' But these days, while far fewer doctors would say those things, they still think like that. It gets passed down from older doctors in med schools teaching residents and it perpetuates the attitude and limits the learning."

In government, there is also limited support or interest. Fortunately, Representatives Yvette Clarke (D-NY) and Lauren Underwood (D-IL) and others are supporters—some since 2007, when still-pending legislation to encourage research into fibroids was introduced.

That's when Representative Stephanie Tubbs Jones (D-OH) introduced a bill to increase funding and awareness of fibroids, especially for Black women. Unfortunately, there were not enough votes to get it through Congress.

The good news is that today there are still representatives who are committed to getting fibroid research funding legislation passed. Representatives Clarke and Underwood and Senators Cory Booker (D-NJ) and Shelley Moore Capito (R-WV) have co-authored a bill that calls for $150 million to go to the NIH for research on uterine fibroids and to support education programs that would help women with fibroids better understand their condition and the treatment options that are available.[7]

"That is why it is so important that we let women in our community know that they are not alone, that we have advocates," adds Valbrun. "Everyone needs to put pressure on their representatives to pass this bill. But however long it takes, it is also vital that we help each woman learn how to advocate for herself with her doctor—and to get the best information and care possible today."

### Increasing Knowledge, Improving Treatment

To advance the understanding of fibroids, Mayo Clinic and its Women's Health Research Center have launched a series of studies.

One is called "A Study to Collect Worldwide Pregnancy Data Following Exablate Treatment of Symptomatic Uterine Fibroids." The Exablate system allows for an incisionless procedure using MR-guided focused ultrasound with thermal monitoring of the treatment effect. The goal of the study is to assess the safety hazards (or lack thereof) in order to support a device labeling change that will allow women who have uterine fibroids and still wish to become pregnant greater access to the Exablate treatment.

A second study is examining the "Cultural Experiences of Black and Hispanic/Latina Women with Uterine Fibroids." We know that almost 25% of Black women ages 18 to 30 have fibroids, compared to about 6% of white women, and they are two to three times more likely to have to contend with recurring fibroids after surgical removal and with complications. Furthermore, 60% of Black women who are 35 or older have fibroids.[8] They are also at least twice as likely as white women to have a hysterectomy. There is very little data on fibroids in the Hispanic community, but we do know they too are more likely to have a hysterectomy than white women. A study in the *Journal of Minimally Invasive Gynecology* looked at the records of more than 1,300 women who had had surgery for uterine fibroids.[9] Only 57% of Black women and 65% of Latina women underwent minimally invasive surgeries, which can preserve fertility, have fewer complications and offer a quicker recovery, compared with 81% of white women.

A third study is on the "Neurovascular Function in Women with Uterine Fibroids." It's focused on the relationship of fibroids in women ages 18 to 50 and high blood pressure: Does one increase the risk of the other? Some studies suggest that around 40% of women with fibroids have hypertension, and others have shown that having high blood pressure is associated with the development of fibroids.[10] It is also known that women who have fibroids going into pregnancy are at risk for hypertensive disorders of pregnancy. It may all have to do with a mix of hormone fluctuations and neurometabolic changes that either condition can trigger.

## ENDING ENDOMETRIOSIS OBLIVION

Endometriosis is one of the most common gynecological diseases, yet, according to Yale Medicine, women in the United States will have endometriosis for an average of 10 years before receiving a proper diagnosis.[11] That's because they don't experience symptoms or their symptoms, such as abdominal pain, are often mistaken for—and downplayed as—menstrual cramps, irritable bowel syndrome and other inflammatory diseases. It is especially common among women in their thirties and forties, and untreated it can cause painful sex, organ damage and infertility.

Women with mild, untreated endometriosis have an unassisted fertility rate of 2–4.5% per month, compared to a 15–20% rate in women without endometriosis. Overall, it may account for 10% of all cases of infertility.[12]

So what is it? Basically, it is when cells that are similar to tissue lining the uterus grow outside the uterus—on the ovaries, fallopian tubes, or throughout the torso. It is thought to be caused by endocrine and immune system dysfunction. It is not a menstrual disorder or disease.

The HHS's Office on Women's Health says that research shows there is a link between endometriosis and other women's health problems, including allergies, asthma, chemical sensitivities, autoimmune diseases, some types of hypothyroidism, fibromyalgia and chronic fatigue syndrome and certain cancers, such as ovarian and breast cancer.[13]

### What We Don't Know

There is a lack of knowledge about why endometriosis happens and how to prevent, diagnose and treat it. And a chronic lack of funding for clinical and lab studies prevents important breakthroughs from happening.

In 2018, the NIH cut endometriosis disease funding to $6 million (which equals roughly $1 per patient). And it just got worse. According to a 2022 study in *Frontiers in Global Women's Health,*

"Research funding for endometriosis is limited, with funding from bodies like the National Institutes of Health (NIH) constituting only 0.038% of the 2022 health budget—for a condition that affects 6.5 million women in the US alone."[14] And the NIH RePORT on funding says that in 2022 just $27 million was allocated to researching endometriosis. In contrast, $278 million was budgeted for research in prostate cancer.[15]

According to the 2023 documentary *Below the Belt,* executive produced by Hillary Clinton and directed by Shannon Cohn, endometriosis—and women's health—is an urgent social justice issue for feminists.[16] To make the case, the film follows the lives of four women living with endometriosis. Some of their comments:

"It just feels like someone is taking a
blowtorch and burning your insides."

"The scariest thing is no one even knows this is going on."

"I found it incredibly difficult to find someone, anyone, who would believe what I said about my own body was true."

"For years, I have been sent to every specialist that makes sense based on my symptoms. They don't see a problem based on their specialty. They don't look at the big picture."

### *Potential Diagnosis Breakthrough*

Imaging tests don't show endometriosis unless it is especially bad. Taking a look using a laparoscope inserted through the belly button has been the only reliable way to determine if endometriosis is the problem—and to excise the proliferating tissue.

But a breakthrough by researchers at Yale and 22 other centers may change that. They are conducting a clinical trial—the EMPOWER Study: Endometriosis Diagnosis Using MicroRNA—of a newly developed blood test to detect endometriosis.[17]

## PERPLEXING PREGNANCY PROBLEMS

"When a woman is pregnant, her whole body changes," says Dr. Virginia Miller, professor emeritus of surgery and physiology and former director of the Women's Health Research Center at Mayo Clinic. "It affects her bones and muscles; it affects how her kidneys work; how she eats; her behaviors."[18] But very little of that information informs how women are treated during their pregnancy, in the delivery room or after birth.

## HIDDEN HAZARDS

For Jaime Richman Comes, relentless pain after childbirth, the cause, long undiagnosed and the symptoms repeatedly mistreated, destroyed her joy at having her first child when she was 42.[19] She told her story to HealthyWomen:

> The pain was unbearable. Was this how every woman felt after giving birth? Since I'd never had a baby before, I had no idea how I should feel. I just knew I was uncomfortable, swollen and in great pain, with no control of my bladder.
>
> I set up an appointment with my OB/GYN but could not tolerate the intense pain when she tried to examine me. I ended up in the emergency room, where they anesthetized me, examined me and

found a vaginal hematoma. The stitches to repair the second-degree tear that happened during delivery had come undone, causing a serious infection. Twelve hours later, I was sent home, happy to be home holding my baby.

Unfortunately, I continued to experience excruciating pain and incontinence. I went back and forth to the OB for several appointments, trying desperately to get control of my pain. Finally, the OB was out of options. With a complete lack of compassion and empathy, she told me, "Expect to be in pain for the rest of your life."

During the next two and a half years, I visited numerous specialists—neurologists, urologists, neuro-urologists, and obstetricians. I was determined to resolve the pain, but all I received were misdiagnoses.

One specialist suggested I see a spine surgeon. Another sent me for nerve blocks, MRIs, three rounds of pelvic floor physical therapy, an EMG (a procedure to test the health of your muscles and nerves) and nine months of acupuncture treatments. Through this ordeal, my mental health suffered.

Finally, after years of disappointment, pain and misdiagnoses, I paid out of pocket to see a specialist who told me that my pudendal nerve was in the middle of my birth canal, and because of the positioning of this nerve, I should have had a C-section rather than a natural birth. Lack of bladder control immediately after delivery was a clear indication of nerve damage. And when I received postpartum surgery for the hematoma, my pudendal nerve was likely cut, causing further complications.

I was referred to a specialist who could perform the unique surgery I needed. In May 2019, I finally had surgery on both the right and left pudendal nerves. It took another eight months for me to recover fully and finally feel pain-free.

I learned that when women experience postpartum pain, it is not uncommon to receive no diagnosis, no guidance, and little support from their medical team.

The range of pregnancy-related health risks that women face because of the lack of focus on their unique physical and emotional needs during gestation and postpartum is truly astounding.

### Maternal Death Risks

According to a 2020 Commonwealth Fund analysis, despite the fact that around 80% of maternal deaths (defined as death during pregnancy and up to 42 days postpartum) are preventable, they've been increasing in the United States—while falling in 10 other high-income countries.[20] In fact, the United States has the highest maternal mortality rate of all developed countries.

Data from the National Center for Health Statistics released in March 2023 showed that there were 32.9 maternal deaths per 100,000 live births in 2021, compared with 23.8 per 100,000 in 2020 and 20.1 in 2019. The total number rose from 861 in 2020 to 1,205 in 2021.[21]

Why? The Commonwealth Fund concluded it is because there's a shortage of care providers—both OB-GYNs and midwives. Furthermore, many maternal deaths happen post-birth, and the United States is the only one of 10 high-income countries that doesn't guarantee access to home visits or paid parental leave in the postpartum period.

Another reason might be the dire impact of COVID-19 on pregnant women, especially Black women, since it increased the effect of social inequities on healthcare. COVID-19 accounted for a quarter of maternal deaths in 2020 and 2021—and the rate for Black women was 69.9 deaths per 100,000 live births, compared to 26.6 deaths per 100,000 live births for white women.

### *Premature Birth*

HealthyWomen has highlighted the increased risk of preterm birth that affects women in the United States. "If you're a woman giving birth in the United States, you're more likely to have a preterm delivery than women in most developed nations," writes HealthyWomen contributor Shannon Shelton Miller.[22] "If you're Black or Native American, the chances of experiencing preterm birth are even higher."

In 2021, a little over one in ten babies born in the United States were preterm—that is, born before the thirty-seventh week of pregnancy.[23] A March of Dimes global map of preterm births[24] shows that the United States has the sixth-highest number of preterm births worldwide, with only Indonesia, Pakistan, Nigeria, China and India reporting more.

### *Who, What, When*

More than 700 women die each year in the United States as a result of pregnancy or its complications. American Indian and Alaska Native and Black women are two to three times as likely to die from a pregnancy-related cause as white women.[25]

According to the NIH's Office of Disease Prevention,[26] around 50,000 women—many of them Black, American Indian or Native Alaskan—contend with life-threatening complications from their pregnancies. These include everything from depression to cardiovascular issues such as blood clots, stroke and heart attack.

Pregnancy-related heart disease and high blood pressure are especially risky conditions for pregnant Black women. A 2021 study in the *American Journal of Public Health* revealed that between 2016 and 2017, pregnant Black women were five times more likely to die from those conditions than white women.[27] In addition, obstetric hemorrhage (excessive blood loss during pregnancy) and obstetric embolism (blood clots during pregnancy) were 2.3–2.6% more likely to kill Black women. Almost all of these pregnancy-related perils are preventable with better pre- and postnatal care—especially for marginalized communities.

With all that isn't known about women's health during pregnancy, it becomes ever more imperative that pregnant women be able to safely enroll in clinical studies.

### The (Distant) Future Is Brighter

The conclusions of the Task Force on Research Specific to Pregnant Women and Lactating Women came out in 2020, and provided advice to the secretary of the Department of Health and Human Services about repairing gaps in knowledge and research on safe and effective therapies for pregnant and lactating women.[28] The findings included:

- "Longstanding obstacles to inclusion of pregnant and lactating women in clinical research studies have limited the collection of data to support the safety and appropriate dosing of medications and other therapeutics used during pregnancy and lactation. While some steps have been taken to address obstacles to this research, such as the recent change to the federal regulations protecting human subjects who participate in research (the "Common Rule"), the culture of protecting pregnant and lactating women from research has proven resistant to change."
- "The presumption that ceasing use of medications throughout pregnancy and lactation is "healthier" for a woman and her offspring is inaccurate in many cases and may actually endanger their health. This danger applies not only to treatments for conditions arising directly from

pregnancy but even more so for treatment of conditions
that occur in reproductive-aged women, whether pregnant,
lactating or neither. Whether women can continue using
their medication for autoimmune conditions, mental health
issues or other chronic diseases needs to be resolved."

• "In the vast majority of cases, the scientific evidence does
not support either continued use or cessation of using
therapeutics, primarily because that evidence does not exist
or is insufficient. Nonetheless, more than 90% of women
use at least one medication during pregnancy, about 70%
use at least one prescription medication and 90–99% of
women receive at least one medication during the first
week after delivery. In addition, many women who become
pregnant or are lactating already have chronic conditions
needing treatment, in addition to conditions that may
arise as a result of pregnancy. Consequently, because so
few studies have been conducted, some prioritization
is necessary to determine which therapeutics should be
studied."

• "Many issues related to the inclusion of pregnant and
lactating women in clinical research studies have defied
resolution for decades, despite efforts over the years to address
them. To achieve this important goal, each of the stakeholder
groups represented on the task force—government, industry,
clinicians and women—has a critical role in carrying out
these implementation steps."

In 2022, the Office of Research on Women's Health held a Pathways to Prevention Workshop, designed to identify risks and interventions that will optimize postpartum health. The goal was to create an

ongoing effort to make evidence-based improvements in postpartum care by identifying risk factors that contribute to poor postpartum outcomes, including social determinants of health (the conditions in which women live, learn, work and play).

I hope that the combination of these various task forces and workshops will help reduce the unnecessary peril that women face when they are pregnant and postpartum. But seeing improvements reflected in statistics about maternal death and disability will take years . . . if nothing stops the forward progress.

### *Rowing Downstream from* Roe

The abortion issue that has polarized the country is a women's health issue—especially when new and proposed legislation does not consider the health of the mother, the fact that a child may have to be carried stillborn for months and then delivered or that women who become pregnant from rape may be forced to bear the child. It is also an issue of a woman's control over her own body and her right to determine when and how she becomes a mother.

Also, revoking a Food and Drug Administration (FDA) certification of a medication, as is being done currently with mifepristone, also known as the "abortion pill," is a terrifying precedent that could lead to arbitrary, medically disastrous impositions of opinion over science. This is playing out in conflicting court rulings, and years from this writing, we may see a Supreme Court decision that could dramatically change the ability of the FDA to endorse safe medications without interference from political opinions.

There is no easy solution to the divisions on this issue, but I am in agreement that you cannot prevent abortions by making them illegal— you can only stop safe abortions. Do you remember back in the 1960s when women would meet someone on a dark corner, get blindfolded and driven to an unknown location for the procedure then dumped back on the street? I do.

Improving education about pregnancy and sexuality and making contraceptives widely available can do a great deal to reduce unintended pregnancies. Plus, providing safe procedures when those measures are not sufficient is the only way to protect women's health regarding unplanned or physically risky pregnancies.

## THE CHALLENGES ASSOCIATED WITH POSTMENOPAUSE

Everything from brain health to immune function, skin integrity, and sexual function may be affected by the transition through peri-menopause (the period before cessation of monthly periods that is characterized by hot flashes, brain fog, etc.), menopause (when menstruation stops) and postmenopause, which can go on for 40 years now that life expectancy, for some women, has increased. Those years may be accompanied by changes in every organ system, the immune system, bone and muscle integrity, and cognition, as well as by the development of dementia and Alzheimer's. The Endocrine Society says an estimated 6,000 women in the United States reach menopause every day.[29]

Changing levels of estrogen and progesterone—and even testosterone—have major effects on every aspect of a woman's body. And that can create challenges for health—as well as for social, economic and familial well-being.

- The SWAN heart study showed that within one year of the last menstrual period, arterial stiffness significantly increased and was greater than could be simply attributed to aging or having other risk factors, such as diabetes.[30]

- A 2021 Opinium Research survey of more than 5,000 women around the world who were experiencing the transition to postmenopause revealed that 60% were adversely affected while on the job, and 33% hid its effects from colleagues and bosses.[31]
- The potential for lost income is also significant. A UK survey found that 59% of women had taken some time off work because of perimenopause symptoms, and 18% said they had taken more than eight weeks off; 2% went on long-term sick leave.[32]

### What's Being Done?

Around three-quarters of the 55 million females in the United States who are experiencing the transition to postmenopause say they receive no treatment for its effects.[33] That is the legacy of the mistaken idea that hormone therapy (HT) (what used to be called hormone replacement therapy) is risky, an inaccurate conclusion that came out of the Women's Health Initiative study.

It is true that these days the American College of Obstetricians and Gynecologists, the American Association of Clinical Endocrinology, and the North American Menopause Society agree that HT is safe for most women in the 5 to 10 years postmenopause, and its risks, even for breast cancer, are minimal. And some doctors are spreading the word. Avrum Bluming, MD, and Carol Tavris, PhD, made it very clear in their popular book *Estrogen Matters* that HT is the most effective treatment for hot flashes, night sweats, insomnia, vaginal dryness, heart palpitations, joint pain and loss of sexual desire, and HT can decrease the risk of death from heart disease in women by 30–50%.

Still, many doctors don't discuss menopause-related symptoms with their patients or prescribe HT, having been educated back when it was actively discouraged or, more recently, simply not having been given instruction on administering it. Mayo Clinic did a survey in 2017 of trainees at all postgraduate levels in family medicine, internal medicine and obstetrics and gynecology at US residency programs and discovered that only 6% of the respondents felt adequately prepared to take care of patients who were going through menopause.[34]

### Sudden Menopause Through Surgery

Another aspect of postmenopausal health involves surgery to remove both ovaries and fallopian tubes in premenopausal women—causing sudden menopause. Around one in eight women in the United States have this surgery, so it is important to know the risks it creates.

The Mayo Clinic SCORE on Sex Differences has focused on understanding how female-specific major hormonal shifts, such as the onset of menstruation, pregnancy and menopause, affect women's cognition and physical health as they age. Currently Mayo's SCORE is conducting three major translational research projects focused on how abrupt endocrine dysfunction, resulting from premenopausal removal of both ovaries, affects accelerated aging and risk of Alzheimer's disease and other brain changes.

Principal investigator Michelle M. Mielke, PhD, is conducting a study on women that is investigating whether removing both ovaries and fallopian tubes accelerates the rate of aging and increases frailty.[35] Another crew of Mayo Clinic investigators is studying whether the removal of women's ovaries and fallopian tubes increases the risk for both Alzheimer's disease and cerebrovascular disease.[36]

"Not all organs age at the same rate and we need to understand how they age in women with their ovaries and fallopian tubes taken out compared to women who experience natural menopause," says Dr. Miller.

To complement those two research projects on human subjects, Mayo Clinic researchers are also using a mouse study to discover whether or not removal of the ovaries affects cell death in the brain and what effect estrogen replacement has on that potentially cognition-damaging effect.[37]

Clearly, there is an astounding amount of information on fibroids, endometriosis, pregnancy, postpartum health and postmenopause that we don't have.

# CHAPTER 10

# Hey, We're Over Here

## Female-Mostly Conditions

The history of all times, and of today especially, teaches that . . . women will be forgotten if they forget to think about themselves.

> —*Louise Otto-Peters, a German suffragist and women's rights activist, 1819–1895*

ritten more than 100 years ago, Louise Otto-Peters's words still apply today. While mainstream medicine has paid some attention to women's health needs when it comes to women-only conditions, aka "bikini medicine," it has almost entirely overlooked the important sex differences in conditions that mostly afflict women. And if we don't think about them ourselves, as Otto-Peters said, they will continue to be forgotten.

## MOSTLY WOMEN, MOSTLY SLIGHTED

Studies by Dr. Art Mirin and others show that diseases that affect mostly women are stepchildren of male-dominated disorders.[1] As noted earlier, Dr. Mirin found that academic researchers and the NIH prioritize male-prevalent killer diseases (not chronic diseases) and allocate funding in ways that favor them. Fortunately, independent healthcare organizations are bucking that trend. "Investigators in Mayo Clinic's Women's Health Research Center are studying why certain illnesses occur only in women or are more prevalent in women compared with men," says Dr. Virginia Miller. "Armed with this information, we are going to become ever-more able to prevent, diagnose and treat women's most debilitating diseases and conditions effectively."[2]

Right now, there are more than 1,400 research studies across Mayo Clinic campuses in Arizona, Florida and Minnesota. Mayo researchers are dedicated to tackling the health issues that continually plague women.

While Mayo's research departments and divisions go from *A* to *U*—from anesthesiology and perioperative medicine to urology—we are going to look at sex differences in the development, diagnosis and treatment of autoimmune diseases and immune responses to infection, Alzheimer's disease, urinary tract issues, irritable bowel syndrome (IBS) and inflammatory bowel disease (IBD), osteoporosis and thyroid diseases. Here's a quick look at just how these conditions impact women.

- Of the 50 million Americans with an autoimmune condition, around 37.5 million are women.[3]
- Alzheimer's affects 6.7 million people age 65 and older in the United States, of whom 4.1 million are women.[4]
- Urinary tract infections and disorders are up to 30 times more common in women than men, according to the HHS's Office on Women's Health, and as many as four in ten women who get a UTI will get at least one more within six months.[5]
- The International Foundation for Gastrointestinal Disorders says that IBS affects between 25 and 45 million people in the United States, and 66% of them are female.[6] That's up to 30 million women.
- IBD—a term for two conditions, Crohn's disease (CD) and ulcerative colitis—affects females (12%) less than males (20%) until puberty, when there is a switch and it is more of a risk for females.[7] Specifically, females age 25–29 and especially those above age 35 are up to 40% more prone to CD compared to males those ages.[8] However, after age 45, men are 20% more likely to have IBD than women. Intriguing.

- Osteoporosis, brittle bone disease in the femur, neck or lower back, affects almost 20% of women and less than 5% of men. And as for osteopenia—lowered bone mass that indicates a major risk for full-blown disease—that affects more than 51% of women and around 33% of men.[9]
- Thyroid diseases, whether autoimmune or not, affect women five to eight times more than men—and can interfere with the menstrual cycle and cause problems during pregnancy.[10] One woman in eight will develop a thyroid disorder during her lifetime.

## THERE'S NO AUTOMATIC UNDERSTANDING OF AUTOIMMUNITY

An autoimmune disorder happens when there is a mistaken attack on your organs or tissue by immune system warriors that are designed to fight off bacteria, parasites, viruses and cancer cells. They are tricked into thinking healthy tissue is putting you in peril and they target it for destruction. We are just beginning to understand how and why this happens—but it appears to be from a combination of genetic and epigenetic factors (the turning on or off of genes); environmental toxins; biological triggers, such as high levels of estrogen in women during childbearing years; infection with a bacteria or virus; a reaction to a medication; and/or even intense chronic stress.

"We know that 75 to 80% of people with an autoimmune disorder are women," says Virginia Ladd, founder, past president emeritus and advisor to the president of the Autoimmune Association (originally known as the American Autoimmune Related Diseases Association). "But we don't really know how many people in the US have an autoimmune disease, since they are frequently un- or misdiagnosed and underreported."

The latest estimate from the Autoimmune Association[11] is that 50 million Americans (37 million women) have at least one autoimmune disorder. However, no one is really sure. Around 25% of those folks (again, mostly women) are likely to develop one or more other autoimmune conditions.

Dr. Frederick Miller, an NIH scientist emeritus and former head of the National Institute of Environmental Health Sciences' Environmental Autoimmunity Group, published a remarkable paper in February 2023 in *Current Opinion in Immunology* that pinpointed just why it is so difficult to figure out how many folks have an autoimmune condition:[12]

- There's a lack of consensus in autoimmune disease definitions, and even in agreement on which specific illnesses constitute autoimmune diseases.
- Many autoimmune diseases go undiagnosed, and variability in certain geographic regions and in ethnic and racial backgrounds makes estimating the total numbers a challenge.
- There are no centralized, standardized databases to collect relevant data.
- There is no coordinated, orchestrated approach to research.

"What we do know," says Ladd, "is that a different way of looking at the category is needed, so we can discover what commonalities there are between the various disorders, and what is unique to each one. One of the missions of the Autoimmune Association is to get autoimmune disorders recognized as a category that includes all the various conditions. Now, most research is disease specific and fails to look at [the] bigger picture. When we see each condition as a part of a larger immune-moderated disease category, then research can look for underlying causes and solutions. And this all needs to be done with an awareness of sex-specific causes and treatments."

As a 2019 *Frontiers in Endocrinology* study pointed out, women's endocrinological changes during puberty, pregnancy, lactation and menopause have a big impact on the immune system, because of interactions between hormones, innate and adaptive immune systems and pro- and anti-inflammatory molecules such as cytokines. All of that increases the risk for an autoimmune response.[13]

### *Boosting Research on Autoimmunity*

For a long time, research on autoimmune conditions has been underfunded. Spending on autoimmune diseases as a percent of overall NIH disease-related costs stayed at 2.6% between 2013 and 2020, while NIH funding of other conditions rose dramatically.[14]

But finally, in May 2022, the prospects for increased research looked brighter. A congressionally mandated review of the NIH's research efforts in autoimmune diseases was done by the National Academies of Sciences, Engineering, and Medicine. Their findings were published as "Enhancing NIH Research on Autoimmune Disease."[15] The report was particularly focused on issues around identification of risk factors, barriers to diagnosis, diagnostic tools, treatments and prospects for cure. The Autoimmune Association sums up the report's recommendations as follows:[16]

- The NIH should establish long-term systems to collect and ensure optimum usability of population-based surveillance and epidemiological data on autoimmune diseases and measures of autoimmunity and support the optimization of existing data sources.

- The NIH should support the development of population cohorts that extend from the period before disease manifests to the development of symptoms and disease in order to examine progression, coexisting morbidities and decade-long outcomes of autoimmune diseases.
- The NIH should provide funding and support for a national research agenda that addresses key gaps identified by the committee.

That led to the December 2022 signing of an omnibus federal spending bill that included the establishment of an Office of Autoimmune Disease Research (OADR) under the NIH's Office of Research on Women's Health (ORWH). In April 2023, the OADR-ORWH was officially established. The stated goals:[17] to have ORWH interact smoothly with already-existing NIH programs and initiatives; to identify areas of research that should be explored; and to improve the lives of people with autoimmune diseases. OADR-ORWH also established the Coordinating Committee on Autoimmune Disease Research, aimed at encouraging collaboration between those with autoimmune expertise.

Now let's see what they actually accomplish.

## SEX DIFFERENCES IN IMMUNE RESPONSES

Autoimmunity isn't the only immune-related health issue that reveals the importance of recognizing sex differences. There are straightforward differences in male and female experience with infectious disease, such as the flu and COVID-19, and in their response to vaccinations.

Martha Nolan, senior policy advisor at HealthyWomen, says that things have improved since 2004, when she asked Dr. Fauci if he ever noticed that there were sex differences in male and female responses to vaccinations. "He was quite pointed in his response to me in front of colleagues of mine. But now we know, from Dr. Sabra Klein's research, that there are significant differences."[18]

### *Males, Females, Flu and COVID-19*

The long-held opinion that vaccines were sex-agnostic has been aggressively debunked by Dr. Sabra Klein. In her 2016 paper, "SeXX Matters in Infectious Disease Pathogenesis," she wrote, "The sexes provide different genetic backgrounds, anatomic niches, immunological profiles, and hormonal environments that can directly affect pathogens as well as the development of diseases following infection. Hormones, genes, and behaviors contribute significantly to sex differences in the outcome of infection."[19]

In her lab and clinical studies, Dr. Klein has shown that premenopausal females tend to develop notably higher immune responses to influenza A and SARS-CoV-2 infections than males. Her studies also indicate that women who get a half dose of the flu vaccine produce as many antibodies as men who get a full dose, and men with high levels of testosterone produce fewer antibodies in response to the flu vaccine compared with men with low testosterone.[20]

"That may explain why men are more likely to contract COVID-19," she says. "They also have a greater inflammatory response to the infection, making them vulnerable to complications and death."

Research out of the United Kingdom and Lebanon has found that in almost all countries with sex-disaggregated data, men are 1.7 times more likely to die from COVID-19 than females.[21] Other studies show an even higher risk.[22]

The sex disparity in the development of long COVID is also telling. A study in *Current Medical Research and Opinion* reveals that when it comes to long COVID, females are more likely to be affected than males.[23] In addition, researchers from the Johnson & Johnson Office of the Chief Medical Officer Health of Women team have alerted the healthcare community to the fact that males and females often have different symptoms of long COVID. Looking at data on almost 1.3 million patients, the researchers found that females often report chronic problems with ear, nose and throat irritation; mood changes and fatigue; and neurological, skin, gastrointestinal and rheumatological disorders. Males, on the other hand, end up with more endocrine disorders, such as diabetes and kidney dysfunction.

Another area of Dr. Klein's research has explored the effects of pregnancy on immune responses to viruses, including the influenza A and SARS-CoV-2. "Having high levels of progesterone dampens immune responses," she says, "and while that helps the fetus, it leaves women so vulnerable to infection." That may be why Dr. Klein has found that pregnancy makes women more vulnerable to COVID-19.

Mass General and Brigham and Women's recent research found an interesting twist on pregnancy and susceptibility to COVID-19: it seems women who are carrying a male fetus have lower levels of antibodies to the coronavirus than women carrying a female fetus, suggesting that the sex of a fetus can affect how a pregnant woman responds to infection by a virus.[24]

The Klein Lab has also demonstrated that age impacts vaccine effectiveness differently in men and women. "We know that in women, as estrogen levels decline—with age—so does the antibody response to the flu vaccine," explains Dr. Klein. Despite declining immunity with aging in women, males still show a greater age-associated reduction in immunity to influenza and COVID-19 vaccines than women.[25]

Although Dr. Klein is recognized for the high quality of her research, she still has to combat resistance to the data. "I exist in the women's health world," says Dr. Klein, "but I have to go get my funding and present my research in the infectious disease world, and there's a lot more I have to do to convince people of how important this information is."

"Up to now science hasn't questioned whether the dose needed changes according to one's biological sex. What if we start to make sex-specific doses and formulations?" she asks.

### SEX DIFFERENCES IN ALZHEIMER'S

Despite a great deal of study into the cause of Alzheimer's disease (AD), there are still no solid answers about what triggers it or why more women than men have the condition. We don't know whether amyloid tangles or tau proteins cause AD or are simply a by-product of the condition. Amyloid tangles are clumps of beta amyloid proteins that form between nerve cells and can interfere with the transmission of electrical impulses and, therefore, of information. Tau proteins help maintain brain structure and function, until something goes wrong and they become neurofibrillary tangles. Some people with diagnosed AD have neither of these supposed markers, and others have one or both of them but don't have symptoms of AD.

There are also theories that AD is not a neurological disease but an autoimmune disorder.[26] And recently, it has been suggested that the reason more women than men suffer from AD is that it may be related to hormone fluctuations, such as the reduction of estrogen during menopause.[27] That generally happens in the early or midfifties, and while AD is most commonly diagnosed in women a decade or more after that, we now know that the disease actually begins (without obvious symptoms) years before it is diagnosed.

### What Else We Know

- AD is the eighth leading cause of death for men and the fifth leading cause of death for women.[28]
- Women make up two-thirds of AD cases in the United States.[29]
- Black Americans are roughly 1.5 to 2 times more likely than whites to develop AD and related dementias.[30]
- Women possess much more of an enzyme that creates tau protein, and they are less likely to clear unneeded tau from the brain, leading to the destruction of nerve cells and possibly the increased risk of developing AD.[31]
- Women who start hormone replacement therapy five to six years after the onset of menopause are at increased risk for Alzheimer's compared to earlier use of hormone therapy, which may be protective.[32]
- Amyloid may be deposited to fight off infections in the brain, and since women are more prone to autoimmune diseases and seem to have stronger immune systems than men, they may accumulate more amyloid deposits than men, and that too may increase the risk for AD.[33]

To expand that knowledge, HealthyWomen's Alzheimer's Hub[34] and their initiative You & Your Brain[35] offer a closer look at where research should be going as the medical and scientific community struggles to untangle the mysteries of this disease. The collaboration produced a video, *The Future of Brain Health: Promising Advances in Medicine and Technology,* moderated by John Whyte, MD, MPH, chief medical officer at WebMD.

Dr. Whyte and I worked together on a Medicare Evidence Development & Coverage Advisory Committee, organized by the Centers for Medicare & Medicaid Services, when he was on the SWHR board and during his tenure at the Food and Drug Administration (FDA). While he was there, he worked with Marsha Henderson, then the FDA's associate commissioner for women's health, and helped launch Drug Trial Snapshots, which provide consumers and healthcare professionals with information about who participated in clinical drug trials (including the inclusion or lack of women as study subjects). They are available for past years at FDA.gov.[36] Today, Dr. Whyte continues to advocate for transparency and inclusion.

"Everyone doesn't agree there is a variability based on sex and gender," he says. "They have not seen the difference. Despite the fact that there is an Office of Women's Health, not everyone believes there is a difference in drug response, for example, or in how AD develops. This is an area that needs much more focused research on causes, risks, and sex differences if we are going to help prevent an epidemic in the coming decades."

### The Good-ish News

Recently, two therapies for AD have been approved by the FDA. The first, aducanumab, known as Aduhelm, is very controversial in addition to being very expensive. It is an antibody therapy that targets the tangles of amyloid beta protein, slowing disease progression. The other, lecanemab (brand name Leqembi), is also approved for early or mild Alzheimer's to delay progression. But there is still nothing to prevent AD or stop it once it develops.

## ABCS OF UTIS

Urinary tract infections (UTIs) are common, especially in women. More than half of women will have at least one UTI at some point in their lives, and 25% will have recurring infections.

Why are women more vulnerable? Because a woman's urethra (the tube from the bladder that ushers urine out of the body) is shorter than a man's, making it easier for bacteria from the vagina and anus to get into the bladder. But greater risk and more vulnerable anatomy don't mean more accurate and timely diagnosis or treatment. A 2015 study published in the *Journal of Microbiology* found urinary tract and sexually transmitted infections in women are misdiagnosed by emergency departments nearly half the time.[37]

According to researcher Michelle Hecker, MD, the study found that "less than half [of] the women diagnosed with a urinary tract infection actually had one. And sexually transmitted infections were missed in 37% of the women, many of whom were wrongly diagnosed with urinary tract infections." Just as shocking, 24% of the women diagnosed with UTIs had no possible UTI-related symptoms documented. And they were loaded up with antibiotics that either had no known effect against UTI pathogens or they were given them even though they had a negative urine test, so there was no reason for them to take the medications.

The misuse of antibiotics is especially egregious given the recent findings published in *Nature Microbiology* that found that when women are given antibiotics to treat a UTI, although it eliminates the disease-causing bacteria from the bladder, it doesn't kill those that may be in the intestines, which allows those bacteria to multiply and spread back into the bladder, triggering another UTI.[38] The conclusion: contrary to what is usually said, UTIs are not caused by poor hygiene.

As one of the senior authors of the study, Scott J. Hultgren, PhD, said at the time, "It's frustrating for women who are coming in to the doctor with recurrence after recurrence after recurrence, and the doctor, who's typically male, gives them advice about hygiene. It's not necessarily poor hygiene that's causing this. The problem lies in the disease itself, in this connection between the gut and the bladder and levels of inflammation. Basically, physicians don't know what to do with recurrent UTI. All they have is antibiotics, so they throw more antibiotics at the problem, which probably just makes things worse."[39]

Again, lack of careful research into the cause and effect of a disease that affects mostly women has meant that women's suffering not only continues but is magnified.

## THE GUTS OF THE MATTER: IBS AND IBD

IBS affects an estimated 25 to 45 million women, who account for almost two-thirds of cases in the United States.[40] It can cause chronic physical pain and social distress and is associated with constipation and diarrhea, but it can't be reliably explained by physical abnormalities or diagnosed by blood tests, abdominal imaging studies or tissue samples.

There is only a patchwork of knowledge about the disorder, and no known ways to prevent or cure it. Treatment depends on hit-or-miss lifestyle and dietary adjustments and the use of repurposed medications, such as tricyclic and SSRI antidepressants and anticonvulsants, such as pregabalin, as well as medicines to ease symptoms such as bloating, constipation and/or diarrhea.

Frequently it is associated with depression and anxiety. According to a study done by the University of Missouri School of Medicine, depression and anxiety are twice as frequent in IBS patients as those without IBS.[41] Over a three-year period, 38% of more than 1.2 million IBS patients that they had data on experienced anxiety and 27% had depression.

### What Causes All This Distress and Discomfort?

One theory is that women's menstrual cycle and perimenopause trigger microbiome disruptions. For example, studies done by the International Foundation for Gastrointestinal Disorders (IFFGD) found that around 45% of women with severe menstrual cramping and 35% of those with PMS also have IBS.[42] And 30% of women with IBS report chronic pelvic pain. But, says the IFFGD, "for the most part the effects of estrogen, progesterone, or their cycle patterns on bowel motility and pain sensitivity remain under-studied."[43]

Another theory is that the gut-brain axis is responsible for IBS symptoms and the increased risk of depression and anxiety. Zahid Ijaz Tarar, MD, the lead researcher on a University of Missouri study titled "Burden of Anxiety and Depression Among Hospitalized Patients with Irritable Bowel Syndrome: A Nationwide Analysis,"[44] has said, "We've long suspected that dysfunction of the brain-gut axis is bidirectional, such that IBS symptoms influence anxiety and depression, and on the other hand, psychiatric factors cause IBS symptoms. Medical professionals need to treat both ends of the axis."[45]

Research out of UCLA echoes that theory on IBS. Dr. Emeran Mayer, an internationally renowned pioneer in research on the gut-brain connection, believes IBS develops from a disturbance of the communication between the gut and the brain.[46] In an article from the David Geffen School of Medicine, he said, "IBS is regulated at the brain level and also at the gut level—through the little brain inside the gut—at the same time. . . . It's actually a loop; it's bi-directional. No matter where the problem starts, it always feeds back and involves the other components as well."

We know women's gut function and biome is distinct from men's in several ways. But I still have a gut feeling it is going to be a long time before we address this women-mostly disorder in a way that allows for effective diagnosis and treatment.

### Inflammatory Bowel Disease: Crohn's Disease and Ulcerative Colitis

IBD includes Crohn's disease and ulcerative colitis. Both conditions are characterized by chronic inflammation of the digestive tract that can cause serious damage to the gastrointestinal system. From age 25 to menopause, women are 40% more likely to develop IBD than men.[47] But men are at greater risk for diagnosis than women when they are younger than 25 and after around age 60. Once again, there is a connection between a gastro disorder, hormones and the menstrual cycle.

Women with IBD are more likely to experience premenstrual symptoms, and symptoms of IBD, such as diarrhea and abdominal pain, are often more severe right before and during menstruation.[48]

In addition, women with IBD may have trouble getting pregnant; if they do become pregnant, some may experience remission of symptoms and some may experience worsening symptoms. There also may be an increased risk of premature birth, low birth rate and the need for a C-section if a woman with IBD becomes pregnant.

## TREATMENT DELAYED, LIFE RESHAPED

It took years for Renika Woods to get an accurate diagnosis of Crohn's disease—and more years for her to find the medical solution to her severe symptoms and an emotional solution to the challenges of coping with this chronic disease.[49]

> By the time I was 27, I was so used to being sick that I knew no other way of life. I had chronic diarrhea and bouts of dramatic weight loss. I was often nauseated and fatigued, and my stomach was on fire with pain. Usually I just attributed the discomfort to stress. But that year my symptoms became so intense that I went to my primary care physician (PCP) for bloodwork.
>
> My PCP informed me that I had a very low blood count. She believed I was passing blood microscopically somehow. She referred me to a gastroenterologist to undergo a colonoscopy.
>
> At first, the gastroenterologist thought I had ulcerative colitis. The gastroenterologist was a nice guy, but not terribly thorough. He merely gave me a pamphlet on ulcerative colitis, a list of foods I couldn't eat (basically anything with fiber, caffeine or dairy) and a prescription for aminosalicylates to control inflammation in the lining of my digestive tract, and sent me on my way. I really wanted the medication to work, but it only made me feel worse.

As the years went on and my symptoms persisted, I practically became a regular at the ER. Finally, in my early thirties, I was diagnosed with Crohn's disease. I started on a new treatment plan that entailed giving myself injections.

That delay in accurate diagnosis had allowed the Crohn's to flourish unchecked.

For a while, I felt better, but then the scariest event of my illness happened: My navel was leaking an odorous fluid. Crohn's just wouldn't quit. No matter how hard I fought, it still found a way to hurt and drain me.

I began to seriously question how I could go on this way. The answer I kept coming back to was that I couldn't. Crohn's would always find ways to make me miserable and in peril. Until I took the most drastic measure: undergoing a loop colostomy. That meant having a colostomy bag affixed to my abdomen, collecting my body's waste.

The thought of losing this core piece of my body, and the image of a colostomy bag, made me feel uncomfortable and vulnerable. But I persisted in educating myself until I had an epiphany: A colostomy wouldn't mean losing control of my body; it would mean gaining control of it after all these years of suffering.

Now I understand that I went through all those trials and tribulations, all those medical conversations and unanswered questions, so that I could become who I was meant to be: a Crohn's warrior.

### The Research Gap

What's being done to push research into IBD and female biology? Not enough. Recently, Komodo Health looked at available data on women's experience with diagnosis and treatment of IBD. They found that despite having a higher incidence of the conditions and presenting earlier with "red flag" symptoms, women not only waited longer than men to receive a diagnosis but, once they were diagnosed, encountered more delays in treatment than men did. In their study population, women made up 57% of new IBD diagnoses, but were only 52% of patients who had surgery and 54% of patients who started taking medications to manage the condition during the month after they were diagnosed.[50]

Another study confirms those findings. Spanish researchers writing in the journal *Inflammatory Bowel Diseases* in 2023 found that compared to males, females with IBD "often experience misdiagnosis and diagnostic delays due to process failures and implicit bias."[51]

And that takes us to the next topic: osteoporosis. According to the Crohn's & Colitis Foundation, 30–60% of people with Crohn's disease have lower-than-average bone density—mostly in the form of osteoporosis, a condition that is vastly more common in women than men.

## OSTEOPOROSIS IS A WOMAN'S CONDITION—NO BONES ABOUT IT

More than half of women are at risk for osteoporosis, and despite the knowledge we have about how to help prevent or slow its development and what can be done to help protect women diagnosed with osteoporosis from independence-destroying bone breaks, there are huge gaps in timely diagnosis and treatment. According to the Bone Health and Osteoporosis Foundation, bone fractures related to osteoporosis are responsible for more hospitalizations than heart attacks, strokes and breast cancer combined.[52] Yet this common, costly and growing problem is often left undiagnosed and untreated.

### Who, What, Why

The World Health Organization criteria reveal that 30% of white postmenopausal women in the United States have osteoporosis.[53] It's often said that at age 60, almost twice as many white women have osteoporosis as Black women, but those stats could be way off because Black women are less likely to be screened for the condition than white women.[54] They also get the short end of the stick if they are diagnosed. Only 8.4% of Black women receive medicine to treat osteoporosis and prevent fractures, and they are 18% less likely to receive medicine following a fracture compared to whites.[55] But even white women are shortchanged: among white women with a 10-year hip fracture risk of more that 3%, only 26% receive treatment.[56]

For all women, the significant risk of developing osteoporosis and having a bone fracture or break happens in part because the transition to menopause is associated with annual bone loss of 4% or more, and that can go on for a decade or longer. Studies of African American women indicate that they generally have higher peak bone mass, but they lose bone mass after menopause at the same rate as Caucasian women.[57]

### A Fractured Future

Cecilia Shouts contends with daily challenges to her quality of life because her osteoporosis-related vertebral fractures were not diagnosed or treated for far too long.[58] As Cecilia told Liz Sauchelli on HealthyWomen.com:

> It had been two weeks since I'd slipped on the front stairs of my home and my back was still in excruciating pain. The emergency room doctor I'd seen after my fall thought I had muscle damage and had sprained my back. He prescribed anti-inflammatories and painkillers without taking an X-ray. At the time, I thought

I was in too much pain for it to be a sprain, but I took his word and went home.

Over the next two weeks, it got to the point where I couldn't even sleep in my bed: I had to sleep in a chair with my legs elevated. My friend convinced me to see a different doctor. The first thing she did was X-ray my back. The supposed muscle damage turned out to be four compressed fractures in my spine. Blood work found I had a severe vitamin D deficiency and a bone density test confirmed I had osteoporosis.

I'd first known I was at risk for osteopenia when I was 27 after I injured my L-5 vertebra in my spine and had a bone density test. Then, at 33, I was officially diagnosed with osteopenia.

But I thought I had done enough to stay healthy. I was incredibly active: I biked, kayaked and walked. In my late twenties, I changed my diet to include foods like leafy greens and beans. I took vitamin D and calcium supplements. Yet here I was at 50 with four compressed fractures and osteoporosis.

After my fractures were diagnosed, I was on bed rest for a month. It then took three months for my back to heal and my vitamin D levels to return to a healthy range. But there have been long-term impacts to my health: Because my fractures weren't treated right away, a curve developed in my back as a result of my broken vertebrae and I shrank 5 inches. I used to be 5 feet, 11 inches and now I'm 5 feet, 6 inches. I can't stand for long periods of time without my back hurting.

I was incredibly upset when I learned that if my compressed fractures had been diagnosed earlier I could have avoided the chronic back pain. What's worse is that the curve shrank the area between my chest and my waist. I try to do stretching exercises to make my stomach more flexible, but there are some days when I can eat three or four bites of a sandwich and I'm full, only to be hungry again two hours later.

That's one of the reasons my misdiagnosis makes me angry: If the ER doctor had X-rayed my spine, I could have gotten better treatment and I wouldn't have developed the curve.

## THE UPS AND DOWNS OF WOMEN AND THYROID DISEASE

We know women are prone to autoimmune disease—and that proves true when it comes to thyroid conditions. For example, an autoimmune thyroid disorder called Graves' disease, which is five times more common in women than men, causes the thyroid to be overactive, while one called Hashimoto's disease, which is four times more prevalent in women than men, makes the thyroid underactive.

More than 80% of patients with Hashimoto's and resulting hypothyroidism (low levels of thyroid hormones) have antithyroid autoantibodies, as well as B-cell and T-cell infiltration of the thyroid gland, consistent with the development of an autoimmune disease, according to a 2021 study in *JAMA*.[59] In a sample of Americans, the prevalence of thyroid-related autoantibodies ranged from 3% of teenage boys and 7% of teenage girls to 12% of men and 30% of women older than 80 years.

The bottom line is that one in eight women will develop thyroid problems during her lifetime. Its prevalence as a "woman's problem" goes a long way to explain why, up until the early twentieth century, thyroid disease was thought to be comorbid with the diagnosis of hysteria. Women with thyroid disease were thought to also have psychiatric disorders that accounted for their fatigue, depression, weight gain or loss and anxiety.[60]

An article in a 1910 edition of *JAMA* stated, "The crying, the laughing, the flushing, the sweating, the rapid heart, the pains without reason, and even the hysterical fever can all be accounted for by reference to the thyroid. The opposite hysterical indifference, apathy, slow heart, hysterical moroseness, and even hysteroepilepsy, may be accounted for by subsecretion, or hyposecretion, of the thyroid."[61]

To make matters worse, since children with mental and developmental challenges occasionally had a mother who had a goiter (from Graves' disease), the prevailing opinion back then was that women with thyroid conditions shouldn't marry.

It takes a long time to shake inbred prejudices out of people, even scientists. A 2018 study in the *Journal of the Endocrine Society* explored the role that sex bias still plays today in the dissatisfaction that women often express about their diagnosis and treatment for thyroid disease.[62]

The researchers found that in their survey of 10,664 female and 502 male respondents receiving thyroid treatment, women were more likely to be dissatisfied with their hypothyroid treatments than men—and a good number were extremely dissatisfied. "Thus," they wrote, "it is conceivable that some dismissal of patients with thyroid disease persists to this day." A recent article in *JAMA Insights* called out the slapdash way thyroid tests are given and interpreted.[63] The authors called for better identification and management of thyroid disease during pregnancy, and in nonpregnant women they said there needed to be more understanding of women's physiological changes, including changes in hormones, at every age and stage so that doctors can optimize the care of women with thyroid disease.

## TOMORROW'S PROMISE

Drug development for conditions that affect women's health has increased notably. A report from the Pharmaceutical Research and

Manufacturers of America, titled "Medicine in Development 2022 Report," says that of the 800 drugs in development for chronic diseases, 625 target diseases that affect women disproportionately or solely.[64]

Now these won't all make it to market—just 12% do—but the medications and treatments that are being considered include:

- 200 drugs targeting cancers that primarily affect women, including breast, ovarian, uterine and cervical cancer.
- 133 drugs for neurologic disorders, including Alzheimer's disease, migraine syndrome and multiple sclerosis.
- 87 drugs for autoimmune conditions, including lupus, myasthenia gravis and scleroderma.
- Treatments for postpartum depression, endometriosis, rheumatoid arthritis and triple-negative breast cancer.

Let's hope these potential advances in treatment options pan out and that many, many more are going to be pursued.

## WHEN THE TABLES TURN

I think it would be ironic—and unconscionable—to not mention one women-mostly disease, breast cancer, in which men are severely slighted. Male breast cancer is 100 times less common among white men than white women and 70 times less common among Black men than Black women. However, for all men, it is often caught at an advanced stage—leading to more aggressive and disruptive treatment and a greater risk of death. For Black men, as for Black women, the prognosis is worse than for white people of either sex. Overall, in 2023 there were an estimated 2,800 new cases of invasive breast cancer in men, and around 530 men died from it. The five-year survival rate for men is 82%.[65]

In contrast, there are almost 4 million women living with or beyond breast cancer in the United States, and it was estimated there would be 43,700 deaths from breast cancer in 2023. But for women, around 64% of breast cancer cases are diagnosed at a localized stage and the five-year relative survival rate is 99%. For those with nonmetastatic invasive breast cancer, it is 91%. Even when the cancer has spread to nearby structures or lymph nodes, the five-year survival rate is 86%.[66]

Men need more attention paid to screening, diagnosis and early treatment so that they are not more gravely affected when diagnosed than most women. Sex differences cut both ways—and this must be recognized.

# CHAPTER 11

## The Great Device Divide

### From the Mesh Mess to Heart Hazards and Disjointed Joint Replacements

It is not the strongest of the species that survives, nor the
most intelligent, but the one most responsive to change.

*—Charles Darwin*

The issue of medical devices and women's health hazards is complicated, since it wasn't until May 1976 that any devices were required to go through premarket review. Officially, they had been "regulated" since the late 1930s, but the manufacturers didn't have to submit proof of safety or effectiveness before their devices were sold to the public. It was President Gerald Ford in 1976 who signed the amended Federal Food, Drug, and Cosmetic Act to provide for the safety and effectiveness of medical devices intended for human use.[1] However, devices that were already on the market but never tested in clinical trials on humans were grandfathered into the "approved" list. Even today, with improved oversight and stricter standards in place, some recently developed medical devices have been cleared for use in humans without up-to-date testing because they are considered to present a minimal risk and are based on Food and Drug Administration (FDA)–accepted devices that went into circulation before 1976.

This short history of the management of devices also includes the formation in 1982 of the FDA's Center for Devices and Radiological Health (CDRH). It was an acknowledgment that it was important to make sure that devices were safe and effective. In the mid-1990s, I was invited to be on a board that was exploring how to improve medical devices. As I recall, I was the only woman on it. Members included representatives from device manufacturers such as Johnson & Johnson, Hologic, Cook Group and Baxter. I brought up the issue that all artificial hips and knees were based on the male anatomy. These industry power brokers just looked at me blankly. It had never occurred to them to even think about that.

I had off-the-record conversations with two members of the board. One board member knew that his company's heart stent worked best in men, and the other said his company's heart valve worked better in women than men. But none of this information was available to the public.

It wasn't until 2004 that the Department of Health and Human Services put together an internal task force to expand innovation in healthcare and speed the development of effective new medical technologies. The professed goal was to promote new ideas and solutions that would encourage innovation of new drug and biological products and medical devices. At the time, I felt it was important to support that effort, and I said publicly how pleased the Society was that they were making medical technology innovation a priority. But it took until 2014 for the CDRH, in cooperation with the US Department of Health and Human Services and the Center for Biologics Evaluation and Research, to issue "Evaluation of Sex-Specific Data in Medical Device Clinical Studies—Guidance for Industry and Food and Drug Administration Staff."[2]

That paper's goal was to improve the quality and consistency of available data regarding the performance of medical devices in both sexes. It also outlined the FDA's expectation regarding sex-specific patient enrollment, data analysis and reporting of study information. It stated: "It is important that the variation in data across sex be considered in both study design and interpretation of study data, unless the investigational device is intended for use in only one sex." Coming two and a half years after an initial draft of the document, it also explicitly stated that it "Contains Nonbinding Recommendations."

Representative Rosa DeLauro (D-CT), our hero in so many of these battles, has been trying to get the FDA to strengthen its oversight of medical devices, especially those that negatively impact women, for more than 20 years. Repeatedly, legislation calling for the release of data that clarifies how a device affects women and men had been left on the floor of Congress. And although some new regulations have been issued, it still remains to be seen how they will be implemented.

We know that devices are going to work differently in different populations and they need to be studied in those populations before being prescribed. Taking a hint from Mr. Darwin, it's time for society, the medical community and industry to be responsive to change and authentically improve their attitudes and actions regarding the development, study and approval of devices.

## THE FACTS, JUST THE FACTS, MA'AM

In 2019, the International Consortium of Investigative Journalists released the "Implant Files," an in-depth look at the regulation of the $400 billion global medical device industry.[3] Using artificial intelligence to tease out sex-specific information, the research in the exposé revealed that 67% of the 340,000 people listed as having an adverse event related to a medical device were women, and 33% were men. It also showed that this did not just apply to "women-specific devices," such as implanted contraceptives or breast implants, but also to sex-neutral implants like artificial hips.

It is vitally important to test implants and devices carefully in women. This allows us to better understand women's experience with medical devices and to minimize complications, such as those caused by pelvic mesh, cardiovascular devices and metal-on-metal hip replacements.

## PELVIC MESH MESS

The use of mesh in women for pelvic and urinary conditions was grandfathered in and resulted (years later) in the acknowledgment that vaginal mesh may extrude and cause vaginal bleeding, discharge and pain, and erosion of the mesh can result in damage to the bladder/urethra, causing painful voiding, urinary frequency, urgency, blood in the urine, repeated UTIs and bladder stones and urinary fistula.

## HEART HAZARDS

A good example of how important sex differences are in devices also can be seen in those used to address cardiovascular conditions.

A 2022 study in the *International Journal of Environmental Research and Public Health* states that "among 123 studies (2000–2007) of 78 high-risk cardiovascular devices, 28% did not report the enrollees' sex. Only 33% of the remaining 92 studies included women, and fewer than half of these sex-disaggregated outcome data."[4] When it comes to implantable cardioverter-defibrillators (ICDs), only 15 of 126 participants in the sole premarket study were women, and although the manufacturer said they would do a trial on women, there's no report of such a study having been done. A subsequent independent meta-analysis showed that among women, ICDs are not particularly effective—they don't reduce deaths from heart disease or any other condition.[5]

Another issue: women undergoing percutaneous coronary intervention with drug-eluting coronary stents are at increased risk for both antithrombotic drug–related bleeding and vascular complications compared with men.

The Advanced Medical Technology Association (AdvaMed) is helping manufacturers and regulators find the will to improve the

SEX CELLS

representation of women in preapproval testing of cardiovascular devices. Tara Federici, AdvaMed's vice president for technology and regulatory affairs, has launched a public awareness campaign with a group of leading women cardiologists to encourage recruitment, enrollment and retention of women in clinical trials of devices. "Even though cardiovascular disease is a leading cause of death in women, women are still underrepresented in related medical device clinical trials. In other words, we have a significant problem—the instances of fatal cardiovascular disease in women and the tools we have to solve them are not being adequately leveraged," she says.

## DISJOINTED JOINT REPLACEMENTS

Metal-on-metal (MoM) hip replacements shed cobalt ions and metal fragments, which the FDA says can enter the bloodstream and cause pain and an increased risk of cancer.[6] According to a 2015 study out of Rush University Medical Center, women are at greater risk of developing complications, such as adverse local tissue reaction, dislocation, aseptic loosening, and revision, than men.[7] In addition, women's gait, anatomy, physiology and hormones were not fully considered in initial designs. That may be why a 2013 study in *JAMA Internal Medicine* that looked at data on 35,140 patients found that women who had total hip replacements had a 29% higher risk of implant failure than men.[8]

Unfortunately, the risks to women were discovered in postmarket studies. But at least the MoM hazard did lead to the voluntary recall of the devices by four manufacturers. In 2016, the FDA decided to require premarket approval (the most stringent regulatory category of the FDA's oversight for medical devices) for MoM hip replacements.[9]

As a result, marketing and sales of MoM devices were stopped and the manufacturers had to go through a process of submitting data to the FDA that showed the devices were safe. Only then could they get approval for them. That has never happened, and MoM replacement devices are not available in the United States. (There are two FDA-approved MoM hip resurfacing devices available.)

In addition, there have been changes in the design of hip replacements so that they suit a woman's anatomy. Gender-specific hip implants mean that the stem, the head and the neck of the implant are adjustable for a woman's size and shape. Previously, if the stem of the implant was too long for a given woman's size, for example, it could cause the hip to push out and lead to pain and even hip failure.

## MORE DEVIOUSNESS ABOUT DEVICES

A 2021 report in the *AMA Journal of Ethics,* "Is the FDA Failing Women?"[10] by Rita Redberg, MD, MS, a cardiologist and professor of medicine at the University of California, San Francisco School of Medicine, and Madris Kinard, MBA, a former adverse events subject matter expert for devices and unique device identification at the FDA and founder of Device Events, a cloud-based software service that uses publicly available FDA data to report on device adverse events, reinforces the previous findings of the "Implant Files."

In this paper, Kinard and Redberg examine the history of transcervical contraceptives, breast implants and vaginal meshes intended for use in women. They look at the negative repercussions of grandfathering in devices that were marketed before 1976 and what the CDRH could do to improve the situation.

The paper took my breath away. In some instances, manufacturers got away with failing to report adverse events to the FDA as required. Bayer's Essure was a metal and polyester coiled device that was put into women's fallopian tubes to block the pathway between sperm and egg.

After it was approved for sale in the United States, women began to complain that it caused allergic reactions and chronic pelvic pain and led to hysterectomy. In some cases it was lethal. Although eventually the FDA required a black box warning on the packaging, a Freedom of Information inquiry revealed that the company had 32,000 complaints about the device that had not been sent on to the FDA. Eventually, more than 39,000 women sued Bayer or hired lawyers over their use of Essure. In 2020, with no admission of wrongdoing, the company settled claims against it for $1.6 billion.

In other instances, the authors pointed out, adverse event reports were made to the FDA but not shared with the public. Silicone breast implants were not allowed from 1992 to 2006, and when newer materials became available for implants, the public and doctors assumed they were not risky—even though there were no long-term studies of the effects of those materials when implanted in breasts. However, as concerns grew, "safety advocates began meeting with the FDA in 2015. In 2018, the agency revealed that the adverse event reports existed but were not made public, despite the mandatory reporting requirement. During a public meeting in 2019, the FDA acknowledged that the agency had received over 300,000 breast implant adverse event reports—20 times more than they had previously admitted publicly. After this meeting, then-FDA Commissioner Scott Gottlieb promised release of all AE reports collected through 'alternative summary reporting,' most of which were released in June 2019."

## WHAT'S BEING DONE

The CDRH "Health of Women Program 2022"[11] has a strategic plan that lays out three priorities:

- Sex- and gender-specific analysis and reporting: This is designed to improve the availability, analysis and communication of sex- and gender-specific information about medical devices so that there is the opportunity to improve the performance of medical devices in women.
- An integrated approach for current and emerging issues related to the health of women: By making sure that all health science programs and initiatives within CDRH are in communication and working together, the organization can improve the overall health and quality of life for women.
- The creation of a research road map: CDRH will create a guide designed to help researchers, manufacturers and government personnel navigate the "medical device ecosystem." This will also allow CDRH to identify resources that can be used to more effectively address what needs to be done to improve the health of women.

CDRH is recognizing that sex and gender differences arise not just in sex-specific devices, such as mammogram machines, but also in devices that were meant for both males and females: cardiovascular devices, orthopedic devices, eluting stents and devices in the neuro-logical space.

AdvaMed is also helping manufacturers and regulators find ways to improve the representation of women in preapproval clinical testing of medical devices and to expand women's participation in clinical trials. "For example," says Federici, "reimbursement, compensation and recruitment incentives for women enrolling in clinical trials need to be modernized. The rules are still interpreted by some institutional review boards as meaning that trial sponsors cannot pay for transportation or childcare for participating women."

We will keep our eye on all the complex issues surrounding devices and women's health and report on them on our websites:

WomensHealthResearch.info
SexCells.info
HealthyWomen.org

# CODA: HIGHLIGHTS FROM 2000 THROUGH 2022

**2000**

- The Society for Women's Health Research (SWHR) received a three-year grant from Aventis Pharmaceuticals that provided enough funding to establish conferences on Sex and Gene Expression (SAGE).

**2001**

- The IOM published the ground-shaking report *Exploring the Biological Contributions to Human Health: Does Sex Matter?*[1]

**2002**

- SWHR received a $1 million grant from Ortho-McNeil to establish the Interdisciplinary Science Networks (ISN).

**2003**

- The IOM issued *Unequal Treatment,* an important first look at the problem of racial and ethnic disparities in healthcare.[2]
- SWHR's fifth annual SAGE conference featured speakers on topics including sexual dimorphism in the brain, environmental effects on development and sex chromosome dosage effects.

**2005**

- SWHR's last SAGE conference was held. The conference looked at sex differences in mental health; the molecular, genetic and behavioral bases of drug addiction; chromosome disorders, epigenetics and disease; and metabolism and energy homeostasis.

- The Organization for the Study of Sex Differences (OSSD) was established.

**2006**

- The RAISE Project, sponsored by SWHR and created by Dr. Florence Haseltine, was launched to create a database that collected information about the gender of researchers receiving scientific awards and prizes from 1981 onward.

**2009**

- The Women's Health Office Act of 2009 was passed. It established—and protected—separate Offices of Women's Health within the Centers for Disease Control and Prevention, the Health Resources and Services Administration and the Food and Drug Administration and an Office of Women's Health and Gender-Based Research within the Agency for Healthcare Research and Quality.[3]

**2010**

- OSSD launched *Biology of Sex Differences*.[4] Arthur P. Arnold, PhD, was its first editor in chief. The journal was funded by SWHR and OSSD.
- The Affordable Care Act was passed, which included the Women's Health Office Act, which protects multiple federal offices of women's health from being eliminated or reorganized without the explicit consent of Congress.

**2011**

- SWHR joined with the FDA/OWH to hold a first-of-its-kind

conference on successful approaches to clinical trial diversity: "Dialogues on Diversifying Clinical Trials."[5]

## 2012

- SWHR managed to get an amendment attached to the Food and Drug Administration (FDA) Safety & Innovation Act that forced the agency to look at how demographic subgroups were represented in trials for drugs that had already been approved, to study to what extent demographic analysis played a role in the approval process and to make this information publicly available.

## 2015

- The FDA launched Drug Trials Snapshots to provide transparency about who participated in clinical trials.

## 2018

- Phyllis Greenberger became senior vice president of science and health policy at HealthyWomen.

## 2019

- The Trans-NIH Strategic Plan for Women's Health Research[6] is issued to advance the health of women through promotion of rigorous relevant research; enhanced dissemination and implementation of evidence-based care; and promotion of training that will develop a diverse and robust workforce, advance science and improve evaluation of research that is relevant to the health of women.

## 2020

- *Moving into the Future with New Dimensions and Strategies for Women's Health Research: A Vision for 2020 for Women's Health Research* was published by the Office for Research on Women's Health (ORWH) in 2010.[7] The ORWH's plan was to advance the understanding of sex/gender differences in health and disease; integrate sex/gender perspectives in emerging basic science fields and translational research and technologies; and foster partnerships to improve translating and disseminating health information. We are still struggling to accomplish these goals.
- Kathryn Schubert, MPP, CAE, became the president and CEO of SWHR.

## 2021

- ORWH hosted Advancing NIH Research on the Health of Women: A 2021 Conference. The key topics were (1) clinical practices related to rising maternal morbidity and mortality rates; (2) increasing rates of chronic debilitating conditions in women; and (3) stagnant cervical cancer survival rates. So many pressing health issues remain unmet.

## 2022

- Environmental risks to women's health persist. For example: Women's exposure to chemicals called PFAs (per- and polyfluoroalkyl substances) in cleaning products increases their risk for cardiovascular problems. Middle-aged women with high blood concentrations of PFAs are 70% more likely to develop high blood pressure than their peers who have lower levels of the chemicals.[8]

- SWHR hosts a webinar on "Addressing Concerns and Considerations Surrounding the Inclusion of Pregnant and Lactating Populations in Research."

## CHAPTER 12

# A Brighter Tomorrow

With the new day comes new strength and new thoughts.

—*Eleanor Roosevelt*

The remarkable people who contributed to this book provide the collective power and energy that are transforming the future of healthcare for women, the LBGTQ+ community, people of color—and men.

They each provide a unique insight into where we have been, where we are and where we need to go in clinical and lab-based research, in medical school curriculum, in everyday medical practice as experienced by patients and in the medical industry—pharma, device manufacturers, vaccine development and hospital systems.

Five of the leaders in this movement have shared their vision of the future, filled with hope and trepidation.

**Virginia Miller**, PhD, professor emeritus of surgery and physiology and former director of the Women's Health Research Center at Mayo Clinic: "In years from now I hope that when an individual goes into a doctor's office they will be viewed as the sex and gender they are and that they will have the cultural aspects of their life that may affect their disease as part of the picture too. I also want there to be research that covers all aspects of how a woman's health changes throughout her life. Being more precise and individualizing who the patient is and seeing how that affects the disease processes in each patient has to improve everybody's health."

**Sabra Klein**, PhD, professor, director of the Klein Lab and co-director of the Center for Women's Health, Sex and Gender Research at Johns

Hopkins: "Tomorrow needs to build on the new insights we have made recently. It sometimes takes a pandemic to get us to sit up and take notice of things that have been hidden in plain sight. What the pandemic did is it highlighted the many disparities. For example, we saw that pregnant women are 42% more likely to be hospitalized with severe COVID-19 than nonpregnant women—and that men are much more likely to be in the ICU and die from COVID-19. There is a lot about a female's immune system that might be detrimental and predispose her to an autoimmune response, but when that ramped up immune response is directed to[ward] a virus, it can be beneficial. We need to understand these dynamics and what is unique to a female and a male. But we are only going to get there by having basic research that identifies the exact cells and proteins that are in play and reveals the reasons that a woman's immune system is more robust than that of a man's. When we know that, then we will be better able to create treatments that are appropriate to each sex."

**Janine Clayton**, MD, FARVO, National Institutes of Health (NIH) associate director for research on women's health and director of the NIH Office of Research on Women's Health: "I would challenge everyone to speak up and out for science. Because if science isn't moving forward, we are moving backward. In the healthcare workforce of the future, we want so many kinds of people contributing to the science of tomorrow. I do believe that science can solve society's problems if we work together."

**Marjorie Jenkins**, MD, former director of medical initiatives and scientific engagement in the FDA's Office of Women's Health, currently associate provost and dean of the University of South Carolina School of Medicine, Greenville, and chief academic officer for Prisma Health Upstate:

We have to face facts: The truth of the matter is we haven't come a long way. We are not there.

The NIH has a $49 billion budget funded by taxpayers. Half the population is women, and they are still not tracking data from funded grants to see if the findings apply to women. Overall, less than 25% of published studies disaggregate their data by sex and gender—or go on to analyze it.

The National Academies of Sciences, Engineering and Medicine [NASEM] (formerly called the Institutes of Medicine), along with thirteen other sponsors across federal offices and NGOs, did that instrumental report with the help of SWHR back in 1993. In spring of 2023, NASEM convened a committee tasked with forming a research agenda around women's health. Thirty years later, there has been a lot of health policy, but it has not had any teeth to it and no established metrics have been integrated into the problem, so that we can measure whether or not the policies have made any difference.

I was invited to present the new committee at the National Academies with a research framework. I told them, "Pick key performance indicators that can tell us where we are NOT and that identify where we want to be in three, five, seven years." You can't measure impact retrospectively, you have to plan, collect the appropriate data and report it.

By creating a research framework that is measurable and with goals the scientific community can commit to, then maybe we can get somewhere.

One area that has made progress: medical school curriculum. I co-chaired the 2016 and 2018 Sex and Gender Medical Education Summit, which was put together by American Medical Women's

Association, Laura W. Bush Institute for Women's Health, Mayo Clinic and Society for Women's Health Research in order to engage educational thought leaders to think about integrating sex- and gender-based evidence into health education. There were virtual summits in 2020 and 2021, with future summits planned.

I am glad to be able to say, we are hearing from a lot more medical schools that they are appointing a director of sex and gender curriculum and building it out across all four years. In addition, the summit has moved sex and gender into a broad array of health professions and disciplines, connecting nursing, pharmacy, dentistry, allied health and medicine.

**Phyllis Greenberger, MSW,** senior vice president of Science & Health Policy for HealthyWomen and past president and CEO of the Society for Women's Health Research (SWHR): I want to add women's voices here as they talk about their patient experience—and give us a clear picture of what we must do in the future to improve their healthcare experiences.

In May 2023 the Kaiser Family Foundation released their findings from a survey of more than 5,000 women ages 18 to 64 who had seen a healthcare provider in the past two years:[1]

- "29% said their doctor had dismissed their symptoms, 15% reported that a provider did not believe they were telling the truth, 19% say their doctor assumed something about them without asking and 13% said that a provider suggested they were personally to blame for a health problem."
- "Just over one-third (35%) of women ages 40–64 say their healthcare provider ever talked to them about what to expect in menopause."

- "One in ten (9%) women ages 18 –64 say that they have experienced discrimination because of their age, gender, race, sexual orientation, religion or some other personal characteristic during a healthcare visit."
- "21% of women (including 38% of uninsured women) say it is difficult to find a doctor who explains things in a way that is easy to understand."

These women deserve better care. It's overdue.

**Marsha Henderson,** former associate commissioner for women's health at the Food and Drug Administration (FDA):

I was so pleased to work at the FDA with brilliant scientists and to coordinate with people focused on sex differences. Advocacy is why things change. And it is more important now than ever.

I am issuing a warning. We are on the precipice. An FDA scientific decision could be reversed, and if it happens, it won't be the last time. What I am telling you now—there are so many areas where things will be stopped.

Did you know that in 2017 the *New York Times* reported there were seven banned words in the CDC? They were *diversity, transgender, fetus, vulnerable, entitlement, evidence-based* and *science-based.* If that's still the case, what do you think is going to happen going forward? We know sex and gender, as issues, are under attack. It is not inconceivable that that could have a chilling effect on separating data by sex. It could restrict FDA approval decisions for all contraceptives, vaccines, fertility treatments and even potential stem cell discoveries for Alzheimer's or Parkinson's disease.

I just want you to think about it. Industry, academia and government have all been moving forward. We don't want to go backwards. We need to advocate yet again. I am saying now is the time to advocate through Congress and other avenues—even if we have to go to the streets. That is the warning I can bring you. Work is going on and it is brilliant work, but we cannot let it stop.

# Hopefully, This Isn't the Last Word

began writing this book more than five years ago, but the struggle for the inclusion of women and minorities in clinical trials has gone on for 30 years and counting. It took decades to convince the National Institutes of Health, the Food and Drug Administration, Congress, research institutions and medical schools that for humans to receive appropriate and effective healthcare, sex, gender, other demographics and geography matter. And it's been an equal battle to see that research on female cells and animals is conducted and reported in a meaningful way.

The reality is that back in late 1990s and early 2000s, I had to convince the American Heart Association that women had heart attacks. They were all about men's heart attacks. The same was true for the National Osteoporosis Foundation (NOF). I talked to the leadership of the NOF when the organization was giving a briefing to congressional staff members and said that they were not focusing on women at all.

I acknowledge that, yes, there has been significant progress in recognition of sex and gender differences since those years, but as the extraordinary research that my co-author Kalia Doner has done and the chapters in this book indicate, there is still a long way to go to understand the implications and incorporate them into diagnosis and treatment.

And while, clearly, improvements that have been made in the diversity of participants in research are important, it's not enough to simply include different populations. It is necessary to quantify and analyze the sex-specific data and use the results to determine the safety, toxicity, dosage and effectiveness of medications, treatments and devices in various populations. That is the front line of the battle now.

It is not a simple process. The more we look, the more differences we find and more questions are raised. It can be frustrating—and very exciting.

When the Society for Women's Health Research (SWHR) was founded in 1990, women's health was thought of as "bikini medicine." It was limited to breast and genital health, pregnancy and conditions such as menopause or fibroids that only affect women. At that time, SWHR was the only organization focusing on sex and racial and ethnic differences in clinical trials. We were frequently rebuffed and ignored (although it never stopped us!).

I recall a meeting many years ago at the Pharmaceutical Manufacturers Association, now known as Pharmaceutical Research and Manufacturers of America (PhRMA). A physician who was a member of the Society's board and I presented our concerns to their scientific committee. Basically, we were dissed. In contrast, this past April, PhRMA announced it was requiring member companies to have diverse samples in their clinical trials.

Progress has been made, but in most clinical trials the number of women included is insufficient to analyze sex-based differences. To increase that number, researchers need to address barriers to participation that women and racial and ethnic minorities face.

- Clinical trials are often held in urban areas. They need to be accessible to women in rural and minority communities.
- In urban areas, information on the availability of clinical trials needs to be brought to the attention of economically and racially diverse communities.

- Researchers need to encourage participation through education and outreach in community spaces, such as churches and beauty salons.
- Researchers need to provide compensation for the additional costs women and racial and ethnic minorities face when participating in clinical trials, such as lost wages, travel expenses and childcare.
- While telemedicine can eliminate some of the barriers that keep minorities and women out of clinical trials, researchers need to contend with the fact that many Americans have no or insufficient internet access.

For this to change, women need to speak out. They need to ask the right questions: Has this medicine or device been tested on women? Do we know if side effects are different in women?

Younger doctors also need to take charge of this issue and demand more attention be paid to sex differences in all aspects of medicine. Hopefully, female and male medical students will read this book and insist on inclusive curriculums.

Outside of the medical, research and social policy communities, other organizations and individuals must actively advocate for more research funding in all aspects of women's health. Contact your member of Congress; make your voice heard.

It's taken over 30 years to get to this point, but we still have a long way to go. We can't afford to wait another 30.

# ACKNOWLEDGMENTS

As we look to the future—and future efforts to improve sex- and gender-specific medicine—I want to thank all the scientists, healthcare policy experts and doctors who were willing to be interviewed for this book. They vividly illuminated the past, current and future challenges of establishing equity in health research and care.

Thank you Drs. Florence Haseltine, Sharonne Hayes, Sabra Klein, Alexandra Lansky, Alyson J. McGregor, C. Noel Bairey Merz, Virginia Miller, Larry Cahill, Kathryn Sandberg, Marjorie Jenkins and Nanette Wenger.

I am also grateful to Dr. Janine Austin Clayton, Dr. Ruth Merkatz and Marsha Henderson for their mighty efforts within the federal government to promote the inclusion of women in medical research and improve how practitioners address women's healthcare.

Many thanks to Mary Ann Liebert, who launched the *Journal of Women's Health* as a result of the Society for Women's Health Research's (SWHR) work, and to Congresswomen Rose DeLauro, whose support was vital to the passage of legislation to establish offices of women's health throughout the NIH and the inclusion of sex differences in basic research.

Other congressional members who were instrumental in requesting the GAO reports and subsequent legislation: Representative Henry Waxman, Representative Pat Schroeder, Representative Connie Morelia, Senator Olympia Snowe, Representative Louise Slaughter and others.

Once again, I want to express my gratitude to Dr. Andrew Pope. Without his support at the Institute of Medicine, the *Biological Contributions to Human Health: Does Sex Matter?* report, which was vital to giving credence to the importance of sex differences, would never have been issued.

My gratitude is boundless to my staff at SWHR, especially to Drs. Sherry Marts and Monica Mallampalli, both of whom were instrumental in increasing sex-differences research, and to Roberta Biegel and Martha Nolan, who led policy and advocacy at SWHR. Monica and Martha continued their work at HealthyWomen.

And a heartfelt thanks to Linda Blount, Dr. Jane L. Delgado, Dr. Queta Bond, Dr. Avrum Bluming, Dr. Carol Tavris, Tara Federici, Virginia Ladd, Dr.

Art Mirin, Dr. John Whyte and Steve Ubl. While the pharmaceutical industry gets a lot of negative reviews, without support and funding from the Pharmaceutical Research and Manufacturers of America and its members, neither SWHR nor HealthyWomen would exist. While acknowledging the importance of conducting research into sex differences has made drug development trials more complicated, the pharmaceutical industry continues to support our work and have been vital to our ability to advocate for their constituents' interests.

I am especially proud that HealthyWomen is continuing SWHR's work by supporting the science of sex differences through advocacy and public policy. It is the largest and most respected women's health organization. I encourage you to check our website. Special thanks go to Beth Battaglino, CEO of HealthyWomen, who is devoted to improving women's health through research, education, communication, advocacy and policy. I am delighted to be part of her team.

I also want to thank Kalia Doner for her extraordinary research, writing and assistance. *Sex Cells* would not have been written without her. And heartfelt thanks to the remarkable team at Mayo Clinic Press: Nina Wiener, Editor in Chief of Mayo Clinic Press, for her support and guidance; Senior Editor Daniela Rapp for her artful shaping of the book; Alan Bradshaw for his diplomatic and precise copy editing; and the remarkable publicity team lead by Jasmine Souers. And I am enormously grateful to all the women who contributed their stories to *Sex Cells*.

The following people were interviewed for the book and contributed to the book with their expertise and insights:

- C. Noel Bairey Merz, MD, FACC, Director of the Barbra Streisand Women's Heart Center at Cedars-Sinai. April 27, 2020
- Beth Battaglino, RN-C, CEO of HealthyWomen, from HealthyWomen's Chronic Pain Summit, healthywomen.org. May 2, 2019, https://www.healthywomen.org/chronic-pain-summit
- Lyn Behnke, a cardiovascular nurse practitioner and Chair of WomenHeart's board of directors. January 8, 2023
- Roberta Biegel, former director of government relations at SWHR. July 19, 2022
- Larry Cahill, PhD, Professor of Neurobiology and Behavior at UC Irvine. January 5, 2022
- Florence Champagne, Chairperson and CEO of the Open My Heart Foundation. November 10, 2022
- Janine Clayton, MD, Associate Director for Research on Women's Health and Director of the Office of Research on Women's Health at the NIH. June 7, 2023
- Jaime Richman Comes, patient interview from HealthyWomen
- Shayla Defils, patient interview from HealthyWomen
- Rosa DeLauro, US Representative. May 1, 2022
- Jane L. Delgado, PhD, President and CEO of the National Alliance for Hispanic Health. March 8, 2022

- Tara Federici, Vice President for Technology and Regulatory Affairs, Advanced Medical Technology Association. January 19, 2023
- Linda Goler Blount, MPH, President and CEO of Black Women's Health Imperative. January 3, 2020
- Soyini Hawkins, MD, MPH, FACOG, founder of the Fibroid and Pelvic Wellness Center of Georgia, from HealthyWomen "WomenTalk: Life with Fibroids, Part 2–YouTube"
- Sharonne Hayes, MD, Founder of the Women's Heart Clinic at Mayo Clinic. May 5, 2023
- Marsha Henderson, former Associate Commissioner for Women's Health at the FDA. April 22, 2020, and November 3, 2022
- Marjorie Jenkins, MD, former director, Medical Initiatives and Scientific Engagement, in the FDA's Office of Women's Health, currently Associate Provost and Dean of the University of South Carolina School of Medicine, Greenville. June 14, 2023
- Sabra Klein, PhD, Professor of Molecular Microbiology and Immunology, Director of the Klein Lab and Co-Director of the Center for Women's Health, Sex and Gender Research at Johns Hopkins. March 25, 2022
- Virginia Ladd, founder, Past President Emeritus and advisor to the President of the Autoimmune Association. January 2020
- Alexandra Lansky, MD, FESC, FACC, Director of the Yale Heart and Vascular Clinical Research Program and the Cardiovascular Research Group. June 7, 2023
- Katherine Leon, patient experience, SCAD Alliance. May 5, 2023
- Mary Ann Liebert, founder and president of Mary Ann Liebert, Inc., publisher of the *Journal of Women's Health*
- Monica Mallampalli, PhD, MSc, CEO of Alliance of Sleep Apnea Partners, former vice president of scientific affairs for SWHR and former senior scientific advisor for HealthyWomen.org. May 1, 2023
- Sherry Marts, PhD, founder and CEO of S*Marts Consulting, former vice president for scientific affairs at SWHR. April 27, 2022
- Alyson J. McGregor, MD, Associate Dean for Faculty Affairs and Development at the University of South Carolina School of Medicine, Greenville, Co-Founder of the Sex and Gender Women's Health Collaborative and a member of the NIH Advisory Committee on Research on Women's Health. May 1, 2023
- Virginia Miller, MBA, PhD, Professor Emeritus of Surgery and Physiology, former director of the Women's Health Research Center at Mayo Clinic. January 17, 2020
- Art Mirin, PhD, a former computational scientist at Lawrence Livermore National Laboratory. March 10, 2022
- Martha Nolan, Senior Policy Advisor at HealthyWomen, former VP, Public Policy for SWHR. February 8, 2020

- Mary Anne Norling, patient interview from WomenHeart
- Andrew M. Pope, PhD, advisor on the Board on Health Sciences Policy, part of the National Academies of Sciences, Engineering, and Medicine, former director of health science policy at the IOM. January 9, 2020
- Kathryn Sandberg, PhD, Professor of Nephrology and Hypertension, Vice Chair for Research at the Department of Medicine at Georgetown University Medical Center and Director of the Center for the Study of Sex Differences in Health, Aging and Disease. November 1, 2021
- Darlene Scott, patient interview from WomenHeart
- Glenda Sexauer, patient interview. September 13, 2022
- Rivka Solomon, patient interview. August 16, 2020
- Steve Ubl, President and CEO of Pharmaceutical Research and Manufacturers of America (PhRMA). April 11, 2022
- Tanika Gray Valbrun, founder of the White Dress Project. September 19, 2022
- Kaveeta P. Vasisht, MD, Associate Commissioner for Women's Health and Director of the Office of Women's Health at the FDA, from "HealthyWomen's Chronic Pain Summit," healthywomen.org, May 2, 2019, https://www.healthywomen.org/chronic-pain-summit
- Christin Veasley, Co-Founder and Director of the Chronic Pain Research Alliance. January 19, 2023
- Lindsay Weitzel, PhD, Founder of MigraineNation and the MigraineNation Patient Navigator Program. January 21, 2023
- Nanette Wenger, MD, Professor Emerita at Emory University School of Medicine, Consultant at the Emory Heart and Vascular Center and Founding Consultant at Emory Women's Heart Center. March 11, 2022
- John Whyte, MD, MPH, Chief Medical Officer at WebMD. March 25, 2022

# NOTES

## PART 1

1. OUTRIGHT International, https://outrightinternational.org/.
2. Andrew J. Webb et al., "Implications for Medication Dosing for Transgender Patients: A Review of the Literature and Recommendations for Pharmacists," *American Journal of Health-System Pharmacy* 77, no. 6 (2020): 427–33, https://doi.org/10.1093/ajhp/zxz355.
3. Deborah McPhail, Marina Rountree-James and Ian Whetter, "Addressing Gaps in Physician Knowledge Regarding Transgender Health and Healthcare Through Medical Education," *Canadian Medical Education Journal* 7, no. 2 (2016): e70–78.

## CHAPTER 1

1. Jean-Baptiste Bonnard, "Male and Female Bodies According to Ancient Greek Physicians," *Clio,* no. 37 (2013), https://doi.org/10.4000/cliowgh .339.
2. Cecilia Tasca et al., "Women and Hysteria in the History of Mental Health," *Clinical Practice and Epidemiology in Mental Health* 8 (2012): 110–19, https://doi.org/10.2174/1745017901208010110.
3. Ibid.
4. Office on Women's Health, "Policy of Inclusion of Women in Clinical Trials," womenshealth.gov, last modified December 17, 2020, https://www .womenshealth.gov/30-achievements/04.
5. Ameeta Parekh et al., "Adverse Effects in Women: Implications for Drug Development and Regulatory Policies," *Expert Review of Clinical Pharmacology* 4, no. 4 (2011): 453–66, https://doi.org/10.1586/ecp.11.29.
6. Alexis Abboud, "Diethylstilbestrol (DES) in the US," Embryo Project Encyclopedia, published March 23, 2015, last modified July 3, 2018, http://embryo.asu.edu/handle/10776/8305.
7. "DES Case Study," in *Women and Health Research: Ethical and Legal Issues of Including Women in Clinical Studies,* vol. 1, ed. Anna C. Mastroianni, Ruth Faden and Daniel Federman (Washington, DC: National Academies

Press, 1994), https://www.ncbi.nlm.nih.gov/books/NBK236538/;
K. Weitzner, J. D. Candidate and H. L. Hirsh, "Diethylstilbestrol-Medicolegal Chronology," *Medical Trial Technique Quarterly* 28, no. 2 (1981): 145–70, https://pubmed.ncbi.nlm.nih.gov/7334927/.

8. The American Cancer Society medical and editorial content team, "DES Exposure: Questions and Answers," American Cancer Society, last updated June 10, 2015, https://www.cancer.org/cancer/risk-prevention/medical-treatments/des-exposure.html.

9. Food and Drug Administration, "Lilly Research Laboratories et al.; Withdrawal of Approval of 28 New Drug Applications [FR Doc No: 00-23477-Filed]," *Federal Register* 65, no. 178 (September 13, 2000): 55264-65, https://www.govinfo.gov/content/pkg/FR-2000-09-13/html/00-23477-Filed.htm.

10. US Thalidomide Survivors, "The True Story of Thalidomide in the US," usthalidomide.org, accessed October 3, 2023, https://usthalidomide.org/our-story-thalidomide-babies-us/#:~:text=They%20were%20wrong.,into%20an%20unauthorized%20marketing%20program.

11. Food and Drug Administration, "Highlights of Prescribing Information [Thalomide]," revised June 2019, https://www.accessdata.fda.gov/drugsatfda_docs/label/2019/020785s067lbl.pdf.

12. Rainey Horwitz, "The Dalkon Shield," Embryo Project Encyclopedia, published January 10, 2018, last modified July 3, 2018, https://embryo.asu.edu/taxonomy/term/38401.

13. Morbidity and Mortality Weekly Report (MMWR), "IUD Safety: Report of a Nationwide Physician Survey," June 29, 1974, https://www.cdc.gov/mmwr/preview/mmwrhtml/lmrk107.htm.

14. Food and Drug Administration, "A History of Medical Device Regulation and Oversight in the United States," last updated August 21, 2023, https://www.fda.gov/medical-devices/overview-device-regulation/history-medical-device-regulation-oversight-united-states.

15. Carol H. Krismann, "Dalkon Shield," *Encyclopedia Britannica,* December 17, 2015, https://www.britannica.com/science/Dalkon-Shield.

16. Florence Haseltine, interview with Tacey Rosolowski, April 9–10, 2016, Renaissance Woman in Medicine Oral History Project, the Foundation for the History of Women in Medicine, https://collections.countway.harvard.edu/onview/files/original/b48075e69723861c33b83f6d8953c78c.pdf.

17. Ibid.

18. National Institutes of Health, Office of Research on Women's Health, "Mission and History," accessed June 14, 2023, https://orwh.od.nih.gov/about/mission-history.

19. Ibid.

20. "Women's Health Initiative (WHI)," National Heart, Lung, and Blood Institute, accessed July 14, 2023, https://www.nhlbi.nih.gov/science/womens-health-initiative-whi.

21. OASH Office on Women's Health, "Who We Are," accessed October 3, 2023, https://www.womenshealth.gov/about-us/who-we-are; Charles Marwick, "Women's Health Action Plan Sees First Anniversary," *JAMA* 268, no. 14 (1992): 1816, https://doi.org/10.1001/jama.1992.034901400 16004.

22. National Institutes of Health, Office of Research on Women's Health, "NIH Inclusion Outreach Toolkit: How to Engage, Recruit, and Retain Women in Clinical Research," accessed October 3, 2023, https://orwh.od .nih.gov/toolkit/recruitment/history.

23. Abboud, "Diethylstilbestrol (DES) in the US"; "NIH Revitalization Act of 1993 Public Law 103-43," in Mastroianni et al., *Women and Health Research: Ethical and Legal Issues of Including Women in Clinical Studies.*

## CHAPTER 2

1. "Veto—or Threat Thereof—Prevails over Majority as 102nd Congress Adjourns," *Washington Memo,* Alan Guttmacher Institute (October 12, 1992): 2–4, https://pubmed.ncbi.nlm.nih.gov/12317790/.

2. Ibid.

3. NIH Grants and Funding, "NIH Policy and Guidelines on the Inclusion of Women and Minorities as Subjects in Clinical Research," accessed October 3, 2023, https://grants.nih.gov/policy/inclusion/women-and -minorities/guidelines.htm#:~:text=The%20NIH%20Revitalization%20 Act%20of,and%20minorities%20in%20clinical%20research.&text=The %20statute%20includes%20a%20specific,and%2C%20in%20particular %20clinical%20trials.

4. "The More Things Change, the More They Stay the Same: A Study to Evaluate Compliance with Inclusion and Assessment of Women and Minorities in Randomized Controlled Trials," *Academic Medicine* 93, no. 4 (April 2018): 630–35, doi: 10.1097/ACM.0000000000002027, https:// www.ncbi.nlm.nih.gov/pmc/articles/PMC5908758/.

5. Philip J. Hilts, "F.D.A. Ends Ban on Women in Drug Testing," *New York Times,* March 25, 1993, https://www.nytimes.com/1993/03/25/us/fda-ends -ban-on-women-in-drug-testing.html#:~:text=Kessler%2C%20said%20 today%20that%20he,they%20became%20pregnant%20during%20tests.

6. Ruth B. Merkatz, "Inclusion of Women in Clinical Trials: A Historical Overview of Scientific Ethical and Legal Issues," *Journal of Obstetric, Gynecologic, and Neonatal Nursing* 27, no. 1 (January 1998), https://www .jognn.org/article/S0884-2175(15)33526-7/fulltext.

7. Food and Drug Administration, "Timeline of FDA Accomplishments in Women's Health: 1993–Present," January 31, 2018, https://www.fda .gov/consumers/free-publications-women/timeline-fda-accomplishments -womens-health-1993-present#:~:text=1994%20E2%80%93%20 Established%20the%20Office%20of,of%20women%20in%20clinical %20trials.

8. Center for Drug Evaluation and Research, US Department of Health and Human Services, Food and Drug Administration, "Guideline for the Study and Evaluation of Gender Differences in the Clinical Evaluation of Drugs," *Federal Register* 58, no. 139 (July 22, 1993): 93D-0236, https://www.fda.gov/media/75648/download.

9. US Public Health Service's Office on Women's Health, *Get Real: Straight Talk About Women's Health* (Washington, DC: US Public Health Service's Office on Women's Health, 1995), available at the Internet Archive, https://archive.org/details/getrealstraightt00unse.

### CHAPTER 3

1. Anna C. Mastroianni, Ruth Faden, and Daniel Federman, eds., *Women and Health Research: Ethical and Legal Issues of Including Women in Clinical Studies*, vol. 1 (Washington, DC: National Academies Press, 1994), https://doi.org/10.17226/2304.

2. Ibid.

3. Institute of Medicine (US) Committee on Understanding the Biology of Sex and Gender Differences, *Exploring the Biological Contributions to Human Health: Does Sex Matter?*, edited by T. M. Wizemann and M. L. Pardue (Washington, DC: National Academies Press, 2001), https://www.ncbi.nlm.nih.gov/books/NBK222288/.

4. Ibid.

5. Mary-Lou Pardue, "Studying Differences Between the Sexes May Spur Improvements in Medicine," *In Focus*, Fall/Winter (2001): 29.

6. "Every Cell Has a Sex," in Institute of Medicine (US) Committee on Understanding the Biology of Sex and Gender Differences, *Exploring the Biological Contributions to Human Health*, 2.

### CHAPTER 4

1. Phyllis Greenberger, "Women and Tobacco Use," *Journal of Women's Health and Gender-Based Medicine* 10, no. 3 (April 2001): 221–22, published online July 7, 2004, https://doi.org/10.1089/152460901300139952.

2. Phyllis Greenberger, "Women, Men, and Pain," *Journal of Women's Health and Gender-Based Medicine* 10, no. 4 (May 2001): 309–10, published online July 7, 2004, https://doi.org/10.1089/152460901750269616.

3. National Institutes of Health, "Women's Health Initiative Reaffirms Use of Short-Term Hormone Replacement Therapy for Younger Women," news release, October 17, 2013, https://www.nih.gov/news-events/news-releases/womens-health-initiative-reaffirms-use-short-term-hormone-replacement-therapy-younger-women.

4. The North American Menopause Society, the American Society for Reproductive Medicine, and the Endocrine Society (drafted jointly), "The

Experts Do Agree About Hormone Therapy," www.menopause.org, accessed September 9, 2023, https://www.menopause.org/for-women /menopauseflashes/menopause-symptoms-and-treatments/the-experts-do -agree-about-hormone-therapy.

5. Office of Research on Women's Health, "Specialized Centers of Research (SCOR) on Sex Differences" poster, accessed October 3, 2023, https:// orwh.od.nih.gov/sites/orwh/files/docs/SCORE_Poster508C.pdf.

6. National Institutes of Health, "Specialized Centers of Research Excellence (SCORE) on Sex Differences (U54 Clinical Trial Opportunity)," due dates August 1, 2022–August 15, 2024, funding opportunity announcement (FOA) number RFA-OD-22-014, accessed October 3, 2023, https://grants .nih.gov/grants/guide/rfa-files/rfa-od-22-014.html#:~:text=The%20 Specialized%20Centers%20of%20Research,interaction%20between%20 sex%20and%2For.

7. Organization for the Study of Sex Differences First Annual Meeting, May 9–12, 2007, schedule of events, accessed October 3, 2023, https://www .ossdweb.org/assets/docs/2007%20OSSD%20Annual%20Meeting%20 Program.pdf.

8. OASH Office on Women's Health, "Creation of Offices on Women's Health at the Federal Level," last updated December 17, 2020, https:// www.womenshealth.gov/30-achievements/17.

9. US Food and Drug Administration, "FDA Drug Trials Snapshots," last updated August 24, 2023, https://www.fda.gov/drugs/drug-approvals-and -databases/drug-trials-snapshots.

10. Departments of Labor, Health and Human Services, Education, and Related Agencies, Appropriations for 2016, "Hearings Before a Subcommittee of the Committee on Appropriations, House of Representatives" (Washington, DC: US Government Publishing Office, 2015), 212, available at https://books.google.com/books?id=cz_5Ns_RBY 8C&pg=PA212&lpg=PA212&dq=Collins+We+have+now+had+extensive +conversations+with+all+of+the+institute+directors,+the+scientific +community+and+my+Advisory+Committee+to+the+Director,+which +is+my+most+senior+advisory+group,+about+this+issue&source=bl&ots =Z_ChQ8_FJh&sig=ACfU3U2_ZkAw03OTE5aAcybWD8z5fdw8nA &hl=en&sa=X&ved=2ahUKEwiD1rjEtLeBAxUtD1kFHZoADDIQ6A F6BAgnEAM#v=onepage&q=Collins%20We%20have%20now%20 had%20extensive%20conversations%20with%20all%20of%20the%20 institute%20directors%2C%20the%20scientific%20community%20and %20my%20Advisory%20Committee%20to%20the%20Director%2C %20which%20is%20my%20most%20senior%20advisory%20group% 2C%20about%20this%20issue&f=false.

11. Janine A. Clayton and Francis S. Collins, "Policy: NIH to Balance Sex in Cell and Animal Studies," *Nature* 509, no. 7500 (2014): 282–83, https:// doi.org/10.1038/509282a.

12. Laura Wronski, "TODAY|SurveyMonkey Poll: Women and Healthcare," accessed September 9, 2023, https://www.surveymonkey.com/curiosity /today-women-and-healthcare/.

13. Emily Paulsen, "Recognizing, Addressing Unintended Gender Bias in Patient Care," Duke Health, January 14, 2020, https://physicians.duke health.org/articles/recognizing-addressing-unintended-gender-bias-patient -care; Clayton and Collins, "Policy: NIH to Balance Sex in Cell and Animal Studies."

14. United Nations Development Programme, "Almost 90% of Men/Women Globally Are Biased Against Women: New Analysis Provides Clues to 'Glass Ceiling'; Tools to Shatter It," news release, March 5, 2020, https:// www.undp.org/press-releases/almost-90-men/women-globally-are-biased -against-women.

15. Anke Samulowitz, Ida Gremyr, Erik Eriksson and Gunnel Hensing, "'Brave Men' and 'Emotional Women': A Theory-Guided Literature Review on Gender Bias in Health Care and Gendered Norms Towards Patients with Chronic Pain," *Pain Research and Management* (2018): 1–14, https://doi.org/10.1155/2018/6358624.

### CODA: HIGHLIGHTS FROM 1980 THROUGH 1999

1. US Government Accountability Office, "National Institutes of Health: Problems in Implementing Policy on Women in Study Populations," July 24, 1990, https://www.gao.gov/products/t-hrd-90-50.

2. US Government Accountability Office, "Women's Health: FDA Needs to Ensure More Study of Gender Differences in Prescription Drugs Testing," October 29, 1992, https://www.gao.gov/products/hrd-93-17.

### CHAPTER 5

1. Cassidy R. Sugimoto et al., "Factors Affecting Sex-Related Reporting in Medical Research: A Cross-Disciplinary Bibliometric Analysis," *Lancet* 393, no. 10171 (2019): 550–59, https://doi.org/10.1016/S0140-6736 (18)32995-7.

2. Tanvi Potluri et al., "Sex Reporting in Preclinical Microbiological and Immunological Research," *mBio* 8, no. 6 (November–December 2017): e01868-17, https://www.ncbi.nlm.nih.gov/pmc/articles/PMC5686541/.

3. Matthew E. Arnegard et al., "Sex as a Biological Variable: A 5-Year Progress Report and Call to Action," *Journal of Women's Health* 29, no. 6 (2020): 858–64, https://doi.org/10.1089/jwh.2019.8247; Janine Austin Clayton, "Applying the New SABV (Sex as a Biological Variable) Policy to Research and Clinical Care," *Physiology and Behavior* 187 (2018): 2–5, https://doi.org/10.1016/j.physbeh.2017.08.012.

4. Cara Tannenbaum et al., "Sex and Gender Analysis Improves Science and Engineering," *Nature* 575 (2019): 137–46, https://www.nature.com /articles/s41586-019-1657-6#Abs1.

5.  Nicole C. Woitowich and Teresa K. Woodruff, "Research Community Needs to Better Appreciate the Value of Sex-Based Research," *Proceedings of the National Academy of Sciences* 116, no. 15 (2019): 7154–56, https://doi .org/10.1073/pnas.1903586116.

6.  Nicole C. Woitowich, Annaliese Beery and Teresa Woodruff, "Meta-Research: A 10-Year Follow-Up Study of Sex Inclusion in the Biological Sciences," *eLife* 9 (2020): e56344, https://doi.org/10.7554/eLife.56344.

7.  Yesenia Garcia-Sifuentes and Donna L. Maney, "Reporting and Misreporting of Sex Differences in the Biological Sciences," *ELife* 10 (2021), https://doi.org/10.7554/eLife.70817.

8.  Arthur Mirin, "Gender Disparity in the Funding of Diseases by the U.S. National Institutes of Health," *Journal of Women's Health* 30, no. 7 (July 2021): 956–63, https://pubmed.ncbi.nlm.nih.gov/33232627/.

9.  US Government Accountability Office, "Drug Safety: Most Drugs Withdrawn in Recent Years Had Greater Health Risks for Women," January 19, 2001, https://www.gao.gov/products/gao-01-286r; Anna Nowogrodzki, "Inequality in Medicine," *Nature* 550 (2017): s18–s19, https://doi.org/10.1038/550S18a.

10. Akshanth R. Polepally et al., "Model-Based Lamotrigine Clearance Changes During Pregnancy: Clinical Implication," *Annals of Clinical and Translational Neurology* 1, no. 2 (2014): 99–106, https://doi.org/10.1002 /acn3.29.

11. US Government Accountability Office, "Drug Safety: Most Drugs Withdrawn in Recent Years Had Greater Health Risks for Women."

12. Geert Labots et al., "Gender Differences in Clinical Registration Trials: Is There a Real Problem?," *British Journal of Clinical Pharmacology* 84 (2018): 700–707, https://doi.org/10.1111/bcp.13497.

13. Irving Zucker and Brian J. Prendergast, "Sex Differences in Pharmacokinetics Predict Adverse Drug Reactions in Women," *Biology of Sex Differences* 11, no. 1 (2020): 32, https://doi.org/10.1186/s13293-020 -00308-5.

14. Marius Rademaker, "Do Women Have More Adverse Drug Reactions?," *American Journal of Clinical Dermatology* 2, no. 6 (2001): 349–51, https:// doi.org/10.2165/00128071-200102060-00001; Flavia Franconi and Ilaria Campesi, "Pharmacogenomics, Pharmacokinetics and Pharmacodynamics: Interaction with Biological Differences Between Men and Women," *British Journal of Pharmacology* 171, no. 3 (2014): 580–94, https://doi.org/10.1111 /bph.12362.

15. Tanvee Varma et al., "Metrics, Baseline Scores, and a Tool to Improve Sponsor Performance on Clinical Trial Diversity: Retrospective Cross Sectional Study," *BMJ Medicine* 2, no. 1 (2023): e000395, https://doi.org /10.1136/bmjmed-2022-000395.

16. Helen M. Pettinati et al., "Gender Differences with High-Dose Naltrexone in Patients with Co-Occurring Cocaine and Alcohol Dependence," *Journal*

of *Substance Abuse Treatment* 34, no. 4 (2008): 378–90, https://doi.org/10
.1016/j.jsat.2007.05.011.

17. Thorsten Buch et al., "Benefits of a Factorial Design Focusing on Inclusion
of Female and Male Animals in One Experiment," *Journal of Molecular
Medicine* 97, no. 6 (2019): 871–77, https://doi.org/10.1007/s00109-019
-01774-0; Cara Tannenbaum et al. "Sex and Gender Analysis Improves
Science and Engineering," *Nature* 575, no. 7781 (2019): 137–46, https://
doi.org/10.1038/s41586-019-1657-6.

18. Jennifer Tsai, "What Role Should Race Play in Medicine?," *Scientific
American,* September 12, 2018, https://blogs.scientificamerican.com/voices
/what-role-should-race-play-in-medicine/; FRAX Fracture Risk Assessment
Tool, "Welcome to FRAX," accessed July 14, 2023, https://www.sheffield
.ac.uk/FRAX/.

19. FRAX Fracture Risk Assessment Tool, "Welcome to FRAX."

20. Davide Cirillo et al., "Sex and Gender Differences and Biases in Artificial
Intelligence for Biomedicine and Healthcare," *NPJ Digital Medicine* 3, no.
81 (2020), https://doi.org/10.1038/s41746-020-0288-5.

21. Deborah Bartz et al., "Clinical Advances in Sex- and Gender-Informed
Medicine to Improve the Health of All," *JAMA Internal Medicine* 180, no.
4 (2020): 574, https://doi.org/10.1001/jamainternmed.2019.7194.

22. Mayo Clinic, *Race and Health: Understanding and Confronting the
Disparities,* special report, supplement to Mayo Clinic Health Letter,
February 2021, accessed October 3, 2023, https://static1.squarespace.com
/static/5e1365b47da94038182d8611/t/6022c6c03f12345e10335409
/1612891841541/Special+Report+with+Mayo+Clinic.pdf.

23. Bartz et al., "Clinical Advances in Sex- and Gender-Informed Medicine to
Improve the Health of All."

24. Ibid.

25. Mayo Clinic Health, *Race and Health;* Andrew E. Budson, "Why Are
Women More Likely to Develop Alzheimer's Disease?," Harvard Health
Publishing, January 20, 2022, https://www.health.harvard.edu/blog
/why-are-women-more-likely-to-develop-alzheimers-disease-20220120
2672.

26. Saion Chatterjee et al., "Type 2 Diabetes as a Risk Factor for Dementia
in Women Compared with Men: A Pooled Analysis of 2.3 Million People
Comprising More Than 100,000 Cases of Dementia," *Diabetes Care* 39,
no. 2 (February 2016): 300–7, https://pubmed.ncbi.nlm.nih.gov/266
81727/.

27. Avni Gupta and José A. Pagán, "Trends in Reported Health Care
Affordability for Men and Women with Employer-Sponsored Health
Insurance Coverage in the US, 2000 to 2020," *JAMA* 328, no. 24 (2022):
2448, https://jamanetwork.com/journals/jama/fullarticle/2799923.

28. New York University, "Health Care Is Increasingly Unaffordable for
People with Employer-Sponsored Health Insurance—Especially Women:

Analysis," medicalxpress.com, December 27, 2022, https://medicalxpress
.com/news/2022-12-health-unaffordable-people-employer-sponsored
-insuranceespecially.html. Dental care: https://medicalxpress.com/tags
/dental+care/; prescription medicine: https://medicalxpress.com/tags
/prescription+medications/; mental health: https://medicalxpress.com/tags
/mental+health/.

29. Alex Montero et al., "Americans' Challenges with Health Care Costs,"
Kaiser Family Foundation, July 14, 2022, https://www.kff.org/health
-costs/issue-brief/americans-challenges-with-health-care-costs/#:~:text
=About%20half%20of%20U.S.%20adults,putting%20off%20due%20
to%20cost.

30. Kaiser Family Foundation, "Women's Health Insurance Coverage,"
December 21, 2022, https://www.kff.org/womens-health-policy/fact-sheet
/womens-health-insurance-coverage/.

31. Caroline Medina, "Fact Sheet: Protecting and Advancing Health Care for
Transgender Adult Communities," Center for American Progress, August
25, 2021, https://www.americanprogress.org/article/fact-sheet-protecting
-advancing-health-care-transgender-adult-communities/.

32. Clare Wilson and Laura A. Cariola, "LGBTQI+ Youth and Mental Health:
A Systematic Review of Qualitative Research," *Adolescent Research Review*
5, no. 2 (2020): 187–211, https://link.springer.com/article/10.1007/s40894
-019-00118-w.

33. Centers for Disease Control and Prevention, "Diagnoses of HIV Infection
in the United States and Dependent Areas, 2018: Gay, Bisexual, and Other
Men Who Have Sex with Men," *HIV Surveillance Report,* 2018, updated
May 31, 2020, https://www.cdc.gov/hiv/library/reports/hiv-surveillance
/vol-31/content/msm.html; Sunday Azagba, Lingpeng Shan and Keely
Latham, "Overweight and Obesity Among Sexual Minority Adults in the
United States," *International Journal of Environmental Research and Public
Health* 16, no. 10 (2019): 1828, https://doi.org/10.3390/ijerph16101828;
Kellen Baker, "Cancer in LGBT Populations: Differences, Disparities,
and Strategies for Change," Presentation, Proceedings of the AACR
Virtual Conference: Thirteenth AACR Conference on the Science of
Cancer Health Disparities in Racial/Ethnic Minorities and the Medically
Underserved, Philadelphia, PA, October 2–4, 2020, https://doi.org/10
.1158/1538-7755.DISP20-IA12.

34. Tyler Santora, "The Confusing World of Breast Cancer Screening for
Transgender People," Breastcancer.org, updated October 2, 2023, https://
www.breastcancer.org/news/screening-transgender-non-binary; Christel
de Blok et al., "Breast Cancer Risk in Transgender People Receiving
Hormone Treatment: Nationwide Cohort Study in the Netherlands," *BMJ*
365 (May 14, 2019): I1652. https://doi.org/10.1136/bmj.I1652.

35. American Association for Cancer Research, "AACR Conference Examines
Cancer Disparities in the LGBTQ Population," January 26, 2021, https://

www.aacr.org/blog/2021/01/26/aacr-conference-examines-cancer
-disparities-in-the-lgbtq-population/#:~:text=Some%20cancers%20that
%20are%20associated,anal%20cancer%20and%20Kaposi%20sarcoma.

36. SAGE, "The Facts on LGBT Aging," 2018, accessed September 9, 2023,
    https://www.sageusa.org/wp-content/uploads/2018/05/sageusa-the-facts
    -on-lgbt-aging.pdf.

37. Leen Aerts et al., "Retrospective Study of the Prevalence and Risk Factors
    of Clitoral Adhesions: Women's Health Providers Should Routinely
    Examine the Glans Clitoris," *Sexual Medicine* 6, no. 2 (2018): 115–22,
    https://doi.org/10.1016/j.esxm.2018.01.003.

38. Helen E. O'Connell, Kalavampara V. Sanjeevan and John M. Hutson,
    "Anatomy of the Clitoris," *Journal of Urology* 174, no. 4, pt. 1 (2005):
    1189–95, https://doi.org/10.1097/01.ju.0000173639.38898.cd.

39. Rachel Gross, "Why Is the Clitoris Ignored by So Many Doctors? Half the
    World Has One, After All," *Irish Times,* October 24, 2022, https://www
    .irishtimes.com/health/your-wellness/2022/10/24/why-is-the-clitoris
    -ignored-by-so-many-doctors-half-the-world-has-one-after-all/.

## CHAPTER 6

1. Cindi Leive, "The First Lady's Quiet Victory," *Glamour,* January 3, 2008,
   https://www.glamour.com/story/laura-bush.

2. Centers for Disease Control and Prevention, "Women and Heart Disease,"
   last updated May 15, 2023, https://www.cdc.gov/heartdisease/women
   .htm#:~:text=Heart%20disease%20is%20the%20leading,in%20every
   %205%20female%20deaths.

3. Keith C. Ferdinand, Herman A. Taylor Jr. and Carlos J. Rodriguez, eds.,
   *Cardiovascular Disease in Racial and Ethnic Minority Populations,* 2nd ed.
   (New York: Humana Press, 2021).

4. American Heart Association, "Heart Disease Awareness Decline
   Spotlights Urgency to Reach Younger Women and Women of Color,"
   September 21, 2020, https://newsroom.heart.org/news/heart-disease
   -awareness-decline-spotlights-urgency-to-reach-younger-women-and
   -women-of-color.

5. Paul M. Ridker et al., "A Randomized Trial of Low-Dose Aspirin in the
   Primary Prevention of Cardiovascular Disease in Women," *New England
   Journal of Medicine* 352, no. 13 (2005): 1293–304, https://doi.org/10
   .1056/NEJMoa050613.

6. WomenHealth and the Society for Women's Health Research, "The 10Q
   Report: Advancing Women's Heart Health Through Improved Research,
   Diagnosis and Treatment," February 14, 2006, https://swhr.org/swhr
   _resource/10q-report-advancing-womens-heart-health-through-improved
   -research-diagnosis-and-treatment/; WomenHealth and the Society for
   Women's Health Research, "The 10Q Report: Advancing Women's Heart
   Health Through Improved Research, Diagnosis and Treatment," June 21,

2011, https://swhr.org/swhr_resource/10q-report-advancing-womens
-heart-health-through-improved-research-diagnosis-and-treatment
/#:~:text=The%2010Q%20Report%2C%20published%20in,of%20
cardiovascular%20disease%20in%20women.

7. Mariana Garcia et al., "Cardiovascular Disease in Women," *Circulation Research* 118, no. 8 (2016): 1273–93, https://doi.org/10.1161/CIRCRES AHA.116.307547.

8. Ibid.

9. Jie Zhang et al., "The Association Between Inflammatory Markers, Serum Lipids and the Risk of Cardiovascular Events in Patients with Rheumatoid Arthritis," *Annals of the Rheumatic Diseases* 73, no. 7 (2014): 1301–8, https://doi.org/10.1136/annrheumdis-2013-204715.

10. Garcia et al., "Cardiovascular Disease in Women."

11. The name is taken from the 1983 film *Yentl,* starring Barbra Streisand, in which her character plays the role of a male in order to receive the education she desires. The phrase was coined by Dr. Bernadine Healy in a 1991 academic paper titled "The Yentl Syndrome." It highlights the distinctions between men's and women's experiences of heart attacks. Bernadine Healy, "The Yentl Syndrome," *New England Journal of Medicine* 325 (1991): 274–76, doi: 10.1056/NEJM199107253250408.

12. Steven E. Reis et al., "Coronary Microvascular Dysfunction Is Highly Prevalent in Women with Chest Pain in the Absence of Coronary Artery Disease: Results from the NHLBI WISE Study," *American Heart Journal* 141, no. 5 (2001): 735–41, https://doi.org/10.1067/mhj.2001.114198.

13. Garcia et al., "Cardiovascular Disease in Women."

14. Olle Melander et al., "Plasma Proneurotensin and Incidence of Diabetes, Cardiovascular Disease, Breast Cancer and Mortality," *JAMA* 308, no. 14 (2012): 1469, https://doi.org/10.1001/jama.2012.12998.

15. Akram Abuful, Yori Gidron and Yaakov Henkin, "Physicians' Attitudes Toward Preventive Therapy for Coronary Artery Disease: Is There a Gender Bias?," *Clinical Cardiology* 28, no. 8 (2005): 389–93, https://doi .org/10.1002/clc.4960280809.

16. Nancy N. Maserejian et al., "Disparities in Physicians' Interpretations of Heart Disease Symptoms by Patient Gender: Results of a Video Vignette Factorial Experiment," *Journal of Women's Health* 18, no. 10 (2009): 1661–67, https://doi.org/10.1089/jwh.2008.1007.

17. L. M. Behnke, "The Danger of Underdiagnosing Coronary Microvascular Disease in Women," *Journal of the American Association of Nurse Practitioners* 34, no. 5 (2022): 780–83, https://doi.org/10.1097/JXX.000 0000000000703.

18. Darcy Banco et al., "Sex and Race Differences in the Evaluation and Treatment of Young Adults Presenting to the Emergency Department with Chest Pain," *Journal of the American Heart Association* 11, no. 10 (2022): e024199, https://doi.org/10.1161/JAHA.121.024199.

19.  G. Martinez-Nadal et al., "An Analysis Based on Sex and Gender in the Chest Pain Unit of an Emergency Department During the Last 12 Years," *European Heart Journal: Acute Cardiovascular Care* 10 (Suppl. 1) (April 2021): zuab020.122, https://academic.oup.com/ehjacc/article/10 /Supplement_1/zuab020.122/6252114; Sophia Antipolis, "Heart Attack Diagnosis Missed in Women More Often Than in Men," European Society of Cardiology, March 12, 2021, https://www.escardio.org/The-ESC/Press -Office/Press-releases/Heart-attack-diagnosis-missed-in-women-more -often-than-in-men#:~:text=In%20women%2C%205%25%20of%20 ACS,initial%20impression%20of%20non%2DACS.

20.  Saraschandra Vallabhajosyula et al., "Sex Disparities in the Management and Outcomes of Cardiogenic Shock Complicating Acute Myocardial Infarction in the Young," *Circulation: Heart Failure* 13, no. 10 (2020), https://doi.org/10.1161/CIRCHEARTFAILURE.120.007154.

21.  Judith H. Lichtman et al., "Sex Differences in the Presentation and Perception of Symptoms Among Young Patients with Myocardial Infarction: Evidence from the VIRGO Study (Variation in Recovery: Role of Gender on Outcomes of Young AMI Patients)," *Circulation* 137, no. 8 (2018): 781–90, https://www.ahajournals.org/doi/10.1161/circulation aha.117.031650.

22.  Norling's story has been abridged, with permission from WomenHeart, from Talia Schmidt, "Champion Spotlight: Mary Anne Norling," WomenHeart, May 1, 2018, https://www.womenheart.org/champion -spotlight-mary-anne-norling/.

23.  Ophélie Gourgas et al., "Differences in Mineral Composition and Morphology Between Men and Women in Aortic Valve Calcification," *Acta Biomaterialia* 106 (2020): 342–50, https://doi.org/10.1016/j.actbio .2020.02.030.

24.  John Brush Jr. et al., "Sex Differences in Symptom Phenotypes Among Patients with Acute Myocardial Infarction," *Circulation: Cardiovascular Quality and Outcomes* 13, no. 2 (February 2020): e005948, doi: 10.1161 /CIRCOUTCOMES.119.005948.

25.  W. Shi et al., "Cardiac Proteomics Reveals Sex Chromosome-Dependent Differences Between Males and Females That Arise Prior to Gonad Formation," *Developmental Cell* 56, no. 21 (2021): 3019–34.e7, https:// doi.org/10.1016/j.devcel.2021.09.022.

26.  Hongwei Ji et al., "Sex Differences in Blood Pressure Trajectories over the Life Course," *JAMA Cardiology* 5, no. 3 (2020): 255, https://doi.org/10 .1001/jamacardio.2019.5306.

27.  Antipolis, "Hypertension Symptoms in Women Often Mistaken for Menopause"; Angela Maas et al., "Cardiovascular Health After Menopause Transition, Pregnancy Disorders and Other Gynaecologic Conditions: A Consensus Document from European Cardiologists, Gynaecologists, and

Endocrinologists," *European Heart Journal* 42, no. 10 (2021): 967–84, https://doi.org/10.1093/eurheartj/ehaa1044.

28. Jacklean Kalibala, Antoinette Pechère-Bertschi and Jules Desmeules, "Gender Differences in Cardiovascular Pharmacotherapy—the Example of Hypertension: A Mini Review," *Frontiers in Pharmacology* 11 (2020), https://doi.org/10.3389/fphar.2020.00564.

29. Muhammad Bilal Tariq et al., "Women with Large Vessel Occlusion Acute Ischemic Stroke Are Less Likely to Be Routed to Comprehensive Stroke Centers," *Journal of the American Heart Association* 12, no. 14 (2023): e029830, https://doi.org/10.1161/JAHA.123.029830.

30. S. U. Khan and E. D. Michos, "Women in Stroke Trials—A Tale of Perpetual Inequity in Cardiovascular Research," *JAMA Neurology* 78, no. 6 (2021): 654–56, https://doi.org/10.1001/jamaneurol.2021.0624.

31. Michael O'Riordan, "'High Index of Suspicion' First Step in Successful Management of SCAD," TCTMD, February 27, 2018, https://www.tctmd.com/news/high-index-suspicion-first-step-successful-management-scad.

32. SCAD Alliance, "About SCAD Alliance," accessed July 13, 2023, https://www.scadalliance.org/about-us/.

33. The Society of Thoracic Surgeons, "Women Undergo Less Aggressive Open Heart Surgery, Experience Worse Outcomes Than Men," NewsWise, January 28, 2021, https://www.newswise.com/articles/women-undergo-less-aggressive-open-heart-surgery-experience-worse-outcomes-than-men?sc=dwhr&xy=10023932.

34. Garcia et al., "Cardiovascular Disease in Women."

35. Nanette K. Wender, "Adverse Cardiovascular Outcomes for Women—Biology, Bias, or Both?," *JAMA Cardiology* 5, no. 3 (2020): 253–54, https://doi.org/10.1001/jamacardio.2019.5576.

## CHAPTER 7

1. Larry Cahill, "Fundamental Sex Difference in Human Brain Architecture," *Proceedings of the National Academy of Sciences* 111, no. 2 (2014): 577–78, https://doi.org/10.1073/pnas.1320954111.

2. National Institutes of Health, "Sex Differences in Brain Anatomy," July 28, 2020, https://www.nih.gov/news-events/nih-research-matters/sex-differences-brain-anatomy#:~:text=Females%20had%20greater%20volume%20in,processing%20different%20types%20of%20information; Torben Hansen, Judith Zaichkowsky and Ad de Jong, "Are Women Always Better Able to Recognize Faces? The Unveiling Role of Exposure Time," *PLOS ONE* 16, no. 10 (2021): e0257741, https://doi.org/10.1371/journal.pone.0257741.

3. Esther Chen et al., "Gender Disparity in Analgesic Treatment of Emergency Department Patients with Acute Abdominal Pain," *Academic*

*Emergency Medicine* 15, no. 5 (May 2008): 414–18, https://pubmed.ncbi
.nlm.nih.gov/18439195/.

4. E. J. Bartley and R. B. Fillingim, "Sex Differences in Pain: A Brief Review
   of Clinical and Experimental Findings," *British Journal of Anaesthesia* 111,
   no. 1 (2013), https://doi.org/10.1093/bja/aet127.

5. Jennifer Tsai, "What Role Should Race Play in Medicine?," *Scientific
   American,* September 12, 2018, https://blogs.scientificamerican.com/voices
   /what-role-should-race-play-in-medicine/.

6. Knox Todd et al., "Ethnicity and Analgesic Practice," *Annals of Emergency
   Medicine* 35, no. 1 (January 2000), https://doi.org/10.1016/S0196-0644
   (00)70099-0.

7. Nicole Sitkin Zelin et al. "Sexual and Gender Minority Health in
   Medical Curricula in New England: A Pilot Study of Medical Student
   Comfort, Competence and Perception of Curricula," *Medical Education
   Online* 23, no. 1 (December 2018): 1461513, doi: 10.1080/10872981.2018
   .1461513.

8. R. I. Klitzman and J. D. Greenberg, "Patterns of Communication Between
   Gay and Lesbian Patients and Their Health Care Providers," *Journal of
   Homosexuality* 42, no. 4 (2002): 65–75, https://doi.org/10.1300/J082
   v42n04_04; A. Westershal, K. Segestenand and C. Bjorkelund, "GPs and
   Lesbian Women in the Consultation: Issues of Awareness and Knowledge,"
   *Scandinavian Journal of Primary Healthcare* 20, no. 4 (2002): 203–207,
   https://doi.org/10.1080/028134302321004845.

9. Weitzer's story is abridged with permission from Danielle Weitzer.
   Danielle Weitzer, "How to Provide Effective Pain Management to LGBTQ
   Individuals," *Practical Pain Management* 19, no. 6 (2019), https://www
   .practicalpainmanagement.com/resources/practice-management/how
   -provide-effective-pain-management-lgbtq-individuals.

10. HealthyWomen editors, "HealthyWomen's Chronic Pain Summit,"
    healthywomen.org, May 2, 2019, https://www.healthywomen.org/chronic
    -pain-summit.

11. Angie Drakulich, "Sex Differences in Pain Response Matter," *Practical
    Pain Management,* April 2, 2020, https://www.practicalpainmanagement
    .com/meeting-summary/sex-differences-pain-response-matter.

12. Lanlan Zhang et al., "Gender Biases in Estimation of Others' Pain,"
    *Journal of Pain* 22, no. 9 (2021): 1048–59, https://doi.org/10.1016
    /j.jpain.2021.03.001.

13. News@TheU, "Research Identifies Gender Bias in Estimation of Patients'
    Pain," University of Miami, news.miami.edu, April 6, 2021, https://news
    .miami.edu/stories/2021/04/research-identifies-gender-bias-in-estimation
    -of-patients-pain.html.

14. Diane E. Hoffmann and Anita J. Tarzian, "The Girl Who Cried Pain: A
    Bias Against Women in the Treatment of Pain," *Journal of Law, Medicine,*

*and Ethics* 29, no. 1 (Spring 2001): 13–27, https://pubmed.ncbi.nlm.nih
.gov/11521267/.

15. Diane E. Hoffmann, Roger B. Fillingim, and Christin Veasley, "The
Woman Who Cried Pain: Do Sex-Based Disparities Still Exist in the
Experience and Treatment of Pain?," *Journal of Law, Medicine, and Ethics*
50, no. 3 (2022): 519–41, https://pubmed.ncbi.nlm.nih.gov/36398644/.

16. Eva Kosek et al., "Do We Need a Third Mechanistic Descriptor for
Chronic Pain States?," *Pain* 157, no. 7 (2016): 1382–86, https://doi.org
/10.1097/j.pain.0000000000000507.

17. A. M. Dydyk and A. Givler, *Central Pain Syndrome* (Treasure Island, FL:
StatPearls Publishing, 2023), https://www.ncbi.nlm.nih.gov/books/NBK
553027/.

18. Institute for Chronic Pain, "What Is Central Sensitization?," March 23,
2013, https://www.instituteforchronicpain.org/understanding-chronic
-pain/what-is-chronic-pain/central-sensitization.

19. International Association for the Study of Pain, "IASP Announces Revised
Definition of Pain," July 16, 2020, https://www.iasp-pain.org/publications
/iasp-news/iasp-announces-revised-definition-of-pain/.

20. Hoffmann, Fillingim, and Veasley, "The Woman Who Cried Pain"; Jo Nijs
et al., "Nociplastic Pain Criteria or Recognition of Central Sensitization?
Pain Phenotyping in the Past, Present and Future," *Journal of Clinical
Medicine* 10, no. 15 (2021): 3203, https://www.mdpi.com/2077-0383/10
/15/3203.

21. International Association for the Study of Pain, "IASP Announces Revised
Definition of Pain," July 16, 2020, https://www.iasp-pain.org/publications
/iasp-news/iasp-announces-revised-definition-of-pain/.

22. A. B. Niculescu et al., "Towards Precision Medicine for Pain: Diagnostic
Biomarkers and Repurposed Drugs," *Molecular Psychiatry* 24, no. 4 (2019):
501–22, https://doi.org/10.1038/s41380-018-0345-5.

23. Rachel A. Schroeder et al., "Sex and Gender Differences in Migraine—
Evaluating Knowledge Gaps," *Journal of Women's Health* 27, no. 8 (2018):
965–73, https://doi.org/10.1089/jwh.2018.7274.

24. Nasim Maleki et al., "Her Versus His Migraine: Multiple Sex Differences
in Brain Function and Structure," *Brain* 135, no. 8 (2012): 2546–59,
https://doi.org/10.1093/brain/aws175.

25. EurekAlert!, "Pregnant Women with Migraine at Higher Risk of
Complications, New Research Finds," news release, June 20, 2021, https://
www.eurekalert.org/news-releases/483557.

26. Bianca Raffaelli et al., "Sex Hormones and Calcitonin Gene–Related
Peptide in Women with Migraine," *Neurology* 100, no. 17 (2023): e1825–
35, https://doi.org/10.1212/WNL.0000000000207114.

27. Martha Nolan, "Let's Dismantle the Obstacles to Treating Migraine
Disease," *The Hill,* June 16, 2022, https://thehill.com/opinion/health

care/3525942-lets-dismantle-the-obstacles-to-treating-migraine
-disease/.

28. Morgan Meissner, "What Disparities Exist in Migraine Diagnosis and
Care?," *Medical News Today,* March 18, 2022, https://www.medicalnews
today.com/articles/migraine-care-disparities.

29. HealthyWomen's information on migraine headaches is available at www
.healthywomen.org/tag/headache-migraine.

30. Committee on the Diagnostic Criteria for Myalgic Encephalomyelitis/
Chronic Fatigue Syndrome, Board on the Health of Select Populations,
Institute of Medicine, "Beyond Myalgic Encephalomyelitis/Chronic
Fatigue Syndrome: Redefining an Illness," National Academies Press,
February 10, 2015, DOI: 10.17226/19012; Ellen Wright Clayton, "Beyond
Myalgic Encephalomyelitis/Chronic Fatigue Syndrome: An IOM Report
on Redefining an Illness," *JAMA* 313 no. 11 (March 17, 2015): 1101–02,
doi:10.1001/jama.2015.1346.

31. Aranka V. Ballering et al., "Persistence of Somatic Symptoms After
COVID-19 in the Netherlands: An Observational Cohort Study," *The
Lancet* 400, no. 10350 (2022): 452–61, https://doi.org/10.1016/S0140
-6736(22)01214-4.

32. Isabella Backman, "Will Long COVID Research Provide Answers for
Poorly Understood Diseases Like ME/CFS?," Yale School of Medicine,
November 1, 2022, https://medicine.yale.edu/news-article/will-long-covid
-research-provide-answers-for-poorly-understood-ailments-like-chronic
-fatigue/.

33. Jaime S., "#MEAction and Mayo ME/CFS Algorithm Is Live!"
#MeAction, April 26, 2023, https://www.meaction.net/2023/04/26/mecfs
-algorithm-is-live/?mc_cid=e71bd1407e&mc_eid=a73e2920b4.

34. E. E. Maher et al., "Ovarian Hormones Regulate Nicotine Consumption
and Accumbens Glutamatergic Plasticity in Female Rats," *eNeuro* 9, no. 3
(June 27, 2022): ENEURO.0286-21.2022, https://www.ncbi.nlm.nih.gov
/pmc/articles/PMC9239849/.

35. National Institutes of Health, News in Health, "How Being Male or
Female Can Affect Your Health," May 2016, https://newsinhealth.nih.gov
/2016/05/sex-gender.

36. National Institute on Drug Abuse, "Substance Use in Women Research
Report: Summary," April 2021, https://nida.nih.gov/publications/research
-reports/substance-use-in-women/summary.

37. Samia Noursi, "Meeting Summary," The Intimate Partner Violence
Screening (IPV) and Counseling Research Symposium, Rockville,
MD, December 9, 2013, https://archives.nida.nih.gov/meetings/2013
/12/intimate-partner-violence-screening-ipv-counseling-research
-symposium.

38. Alicia A. Jacobs and Michelle Cangiano, "Medication-Assisted Treatment
Considerations for Women with Opiate Addiction Disorders," *Primary*

*Care: Clinics in Office Practice* 45, no. 4 (2018): 731–42, https://doi.org
/10.1016/j.pop.2018.08.002; Shelly F. Greenfield et al., "Group Process
in the Single-Gender Women's Recovery Group Compared with Mixed-
Gender Group Drug Counseling," *Journal of Groups in Addiction and
Recovery* 8, no. 4 (2013): 270–93, https://doi.org/10.1080/1556035X
.2013.836867; Tara Lyons et al., "A Qualitative Study of Transgender
Individuals' Experiences in Residential Addiction Treatment Settings:
Stigma and Inclusivity," *Substance Abuse Treatment, Prevention and Policy*
10, no. 1 (2015): 17, https://doi.org/10.1186/s13011-015-0015-4.

39. National Institute on Drug Abuse, "Substance Use in Women Research
Report: Summary." nida.nih.gov/node/22237.

40. Food and Drug Administration, "Executive Summary: Opioid and
Nicotine Use, Dependence and Recovery: Influences of Sex and Gender,"
Opioid and Nicotine Use, Dependence and Recovery: Influences of Sex
and Gender Conference, Silver Spring, MD, September 27–28, 2018,
https://www.fda.gov/media/129282/download?attachment.

## CHAPTER 8

1. Jennifer Niven, *All the Bright Places* (New York: Ember, 2015).

2. Debra J. Brody, Laura A. Pratt and Jeffery P. Hughes, "Prevalence of
Depression Among Adults Aged 20 and Over: United States, 2013–2016,"
NCHS Data Brief, no 303, Hyattsville, MD: National Center for Health
Statistics, 2018, https://www.cdc.gov/nchs/products/databriefs/db303
.htm#:~:text=Overall%2C%20women%20(10.4%25)%20were,differ%20
statistically%20across%20age%20groups.

3. Oriana Vesga-López et al., "Gender Differences in Generalized Anxiety
Disorder: Results from the National Epidemiologic Survey on Alcohol and
Related Conditions (NESARC)," *Journal of Clinical Psychiatry* 69, no. 10
(October 2008): 1606–16, published online September 23, 2008, https://
www.ncbi.nlm.nih.gov/pmc/articles/PMC4765378/#:~:text=Data%20
from%20epidemiological%20studies%20indicate,epidemiology%20of
%20GAD%20by%20gender.

4. Marija Kundakovic and Devin Rocks, "Sex Hormone Fluctuation and
Increased Female Risk for Depression and Anxiety Disorders: From
Clinical Evidence to Molecular Mechanisms," *Frontiers in Neuro-
endocrinology* 66 (2022): 101010, https://doi.org/10.1016/j.yfrne.2022
.101010.

5. Clinical Topics in Depression, "Is Depression Different in Men and
Women?," editorially reviewed by Michael Banov, clinicaltopicsdepression
.com, October 21, 2022, https://www.clinicaltopicsdepression.com
/learning_objectives/depression-different-men-and-women; D. A. Zhukov
and E. P. Vinogradova, "Neurosteroids and Depression," *Neurochemical
Journal* 15, no. 3 (2021): 240–46, https://doi.org/10.1134/S1819712421
030144.

6.  S. Misri, J. Abizadeh, S. Sanders and E. Swift, "Perinatal Generalized Anxiety Disorder: Assessment and Treatment," *Journal of Women's Health* 24, no. 9 (September 1, 2015): 762–70, doi: 10.1089/jwh.2014 .5150, https://www.ncbi.nlm.nih.gov/pmc/articles/PMC4589308/#:~: text=Prevalence%20of%20GAD%20during%20pregnancy,(1.2%25%20 to%206.4%25).

7.  N. Dubey et al., "The ESC/E(Z) Complex, an Effector of Response to Ovarian Steroids, Manifests an Intrinsic Difference in Cells from Women with Premenstrual Dysphoric Disorder," *Molecular Psychiatry* 22, no. 8 (2017): 1172–84, https://doi.org/10.1038/mp.2016.229; National Institutes of Health, "Sex Hormone-Sensitive Gene Complex Linked to Premenstrual Mood Disorder," news release, January 3, 2017, https://www .nih.gov/news-events/news-releases/sex-hormone-sensitive-gene-complex -linked-premenstrual-mood-disorder.

8.  Patrícia Pelufo Silveira et al., "A Sex-Specific Genome-Wide Association Study of Depression Phenotypes in UK Biobank," *Molecular Psychology* (2023), https://doi.org/10.1038/s41380-023-01960-0.

9.  John Elflein, "U.S. Adults with Anxiety Disorder Symptoms from Apr. 2020–Aug. 2023, by Gender," Statista, August 30, 2023, https://www .statista.com/statistics/1132661/anxiety-symptoms-us-adults-by-gender -past-week/.

10.  Office on Women's Health, "Stress and Your Health," accessed September 9, 2023, https://www.womenshealth.gov/mental-health/good-mental -health/stress-and-your-health.

11.  John J. Sramek, Michael F. Murphy and Neal R. Cutler, "Sex Differences in the Psychopharmacological Treatment of Depression," *Dialogues in Clinical Neuroscience* 18, no. 4 (December 2016): 447–57, https://www .ncbi.nlm.nih.gov/pmc/articles/PMC5286730/.

12.  Roni Jacobson, "Psychotropic Drugs Affect Men and Women Differently," *Scientific American,* July 1, 2014, https://www.scientificamerican.com /article/psychotropic-drugs-affect-men-and-women-differently/.

13.  Nanette K. Wenger et al., "Call to Action for Cardiovascular Disease in Women: Epidemiology, Awareness, Access, and Delivery of Equitable Health Care: A Presidential Advisory from the American Heart Association," *Circulation* 145, no. 23 (2022), https://doi.org/10.1161 /CIR.0000000000001071.

### CODA: FINDING RELIEF

1.  The Foundation for Art and Healing, www.ArtandHealing.org.

### CHAPTER 9

1.  Johns Hopkins Medicine, "Fibroids," accessed July 14, 2023, https://www .hopkinsmedicine.org/health/conditions-and-diseases/uterine-fibroids#:~:

text=In%20some%20cases%2C%20fibroids%20can,sometime%20during %20their%20childbearing%20years.

2. Office on Women's Health, "Endometriosis," accessed September 9, 2023, https://www.womenshealth.gov/a-z-topics/endometriosis#:~:text =Endometriosis%20happens%20when%20tissue%20similar,women%20 between%2015%20and%2044.&text=It%20is%20especially%20 common%20among,it%20harder%20to%20get%20pregnant.

3. Sally C. Curtin et al., "Pregnancy Rates for U.S. Women Continue to Drop," NCHS data brief, no. 136, National Center for Health Statistics, 2013, https://www.cdc.gov/nchs/products/databriefs/db136.htm#:~:text =The%20estimated%20number%20of%20pregnancies,2007%20has%20 been%20well%20documented.

4. Elizabeth Chuck, "'No Question' That U.S. Maternal Mortality Rate Will Rise Post-Roe, Experts Say," NBC News, June 30, 2022, https:// www.nbcnews.com/news/us-news/no-question-us-maternal-mortality -rate-will-rise-post-roe-experts-say-rcna35741; Mary Kekatos, "Majority of OB-GYNs Believe Overturning Roe Led to More Maternal Deaths: Survey," ABC News, June 21, 2023, https://abcnews.go.com/Health /majority-obgyns-overturning-roe-led-maternal-deaths-survey/story?id =100241112.

5. M.D. Grant et al., "Menopausal Symptoms: Comparative Effectiveness of Therapies," Agency for Healthcare Research and Quality, *Comparative Effectiveness Reviews,* no. 147 (March 2015), https://www.ncbi.nlm.nih.gov /books/NBK285446/#:~:text=During%20menopause%2C%20 approximately%2085%20percent,of%20varying%20type%20and%20 severity.&text=Types%20of%20symptoms%20experienced%20include %20the%20following.&text=Vasomotor%20symptoms%20are%20 recurrent%2C%20transient,body%2C%20sometimes%20followed%20 by%20chills.

6. Tune into HealthyWomen's videos *Life with Fibroids, Part 1 and Part 2* at healthywomen.org for more information and insights from Dr. Hawkins and Shayla, https://www.youtube.com/watch?v=Hn2GYVz7G6k &feature=youtu.be.

7. Katharine L. Krol, Julie C. Bulman and Judi Buckalew, "IR Legislation," *IR Quarterly,* January 25, 2023, https://irq.sirweb.org/advocacy/ir -legislation/.

8. Beata Mostafavi, "Understanding Racial Disparities for Women with Uterine Fibroids," Michigan Medicine, August 12, 2020, https://www .michiganmedicine.org/health-lab/understanding-racial-disparities -women-uterine-fibroids; Laura Schmidt, "Latinas, Black Women Less Likely to Get Minimally Invasive Fibroid Surgery," TuSalud, September 9, 2022, https://www.tusaludmag.com/article/latinas-black-women-less -likely-get-minimally-invasive-fibroid-surgery.

9. Rebecca Schneyer et al., "The Impact of Race and Ethnicity on Use of Minimally Invasive Surgery for Myomas," *Journal of Minimally Invasive Gynecology* 29, no. 11 (July 3, 2022): 1241–47, https://doi.org/10.1016 /j.jmig.2022.06.025.

10. Yequn Chen et al., "Uterine Fibroids Increase the Risk of Hypertensive Disorders of Pregnancy: A Prospective Cohort Study," *Journal of Hypertension* 39, no. 5 (2021): 1002–8, https://doi.org/10.1097/HJH.000 0000000002729.

11. Yale Medicine, "Endometriosis," accessed September 9, 2023, https:// www.yalemedicine.org/conditions/endometriosis?fbclid=IwAR1I3q5 D8KRviGg9BuEcGKES_l8m2yTHLfJFlWeSHLdVHbobA8T4Dt UdysY.

12. Anis Fadhlaoui, Jean Bouquet de la Joliniere and Anis Feki, "Endometriosis and Infertility: How and When to Treat?," *Frontiers in Surgery* 1 (2014), https://doi.org/10.3389/fsurg.2014.00024.

13. Office on Women's Health, "Endometriosis," accessed September 9, 2023, https://www.womenshealth.gov/a-z-topics/endometriosis.

14. Katherine Ellis, Deborah Munro and Jennifer Clarke, "Endometriosis Is Undervalued: A Call to Action," *Frontiers in Global Women's Health* 3 (2022), https://doi.org/10.3389/fgwh.2022.902371.

15. "Estimates of Funding for Various Research, Condition, and Disease Categories (RCDC)," NIH RePORT, table published March 31, 2023, https://report.nih.gov/funding/categorical-spending#/.

16. *Below the Belt,* directed by Shannon Cohn (RIPP Entertainment Films, 2023).

17. "The EMPOWER Study: Endometriosis Diagnosis Using MicroRNA (EMPOWER)," clinicaltrials.gov, accessed September 9, 2023, https:// classic.clinicaltrials.gov/ct2/show/NCT04598698; Yale Medicine, "Endometriosis."

18. Mayo Clinic, "Women's Health Research Center," accessed July 14, 2023, https://www.mayo.edu/research/centers-programs/womens-health -research-center/overview.

19. Comes's story abridged, with permission from HealthyWomen, from HealthyWomen editors, "I Thought My Postpartum Pain Was Normal, But It Wasn't," HealthyWomen, June 3, 2020, https://www.healthy women.org/content/article/i-thought-my-postpartum-pain-was-normal-it -wasnt.

20. Roosa Tikkanen et al., "Maternal Mortality and Maternity Care in the United States Compared to 10 Other Developed Countries," Commonwealth Fund, November 18, 2020, https://www.common wealthfund.org/publications/issue-briefs/2020/nov/maternal-mortality -maternity-care-us-compared-10-countries; Rachel Diamond, "More Than 4 in 5 Pregnancy-Related Deaths Are Preventable in the US and Mental Health Is the Leading Cause," NewsWise, November 30, 2022, https://

www.newswise.com/articles/more-than-4-in-5-pregnancy-related-deaths
-are-preventable-in-the-us-and-mental-health-is-the-leading-cause?sc
=mwhr&xy=10023932.

21. Donna L. Hoyert, "Maternal Mortality Rates in the United States, 2021,"
NCHS Health E-Stats, 2023, https://www.cdc.gov/nchs/data/hestat
/maternal-mortality/2021/maternal-mortality-rates-2021.htm; Emily
Harris, "US Maternal Mortality Continues to Worsen," *JAMA* 329 no. 15
(2023): 1248, doi:10.1001/jama.2023.5254.

22. Shannon Shelton Miller, "Can Living in the US Increase Your Risk of
Preterm Birth?," HealthyWomen, November 16, 2022, https://www
.healthywomen.org/your-health/us-increase-your-risk-of-preterm-birth.

23. Centers for Disease Control and Prevention, "Preterm Birth," last updated
November 1, 2022, https://www.cdc.gov/reproductivehealth/maternal
infanthealth/pretermbirth.htm.

24. March of Dimes, "Born Too Soon," infographic, accessed October 3,
2023, https://onprem.marchofdimes.org/mission/global-preterm.aspx.

25. National Institutes of Health, Office of Disease Prevention, "Identifying
Risks and Interventions to Optimize Postpartum Health" workshop,
Pathways to Prevention, November 29–December 1, 2022, https://
prevention.nih.gov/research-priorities/research-needs-and-gaps/pathways
-prevention/identifying-risks-and-interventions-optimize-postpartum
-health; Diamond, "More Than 4 in 5 Pregnancy-Related Deaths Are
Preventable in the US, and Mental Health Is the Leading Cause."

26. NIH Office of Disease Prevention, "Pathways to Prevention (P2P)
Program: Identifying Risks and Interventions to Optimize Postpartum
Health," accessed October 3, 2023, https://prevention.nih.gov/research
-priorities/research-needs-and-gaps/pathways-prevention/identifying
-risks-and-interventions-optimize-postpartum-health.

27. Marian MacDorman et al., "Racial and Ethnic Disparities in Maternal
Mortality in the United States Using Enhanced Vital Records, 2016–
2017," *American Journal of Public Health* 111 no. 9 (September 1, 2021):
1673–81, https://ajph.aphapublications.org/doi/full/10.2105/AJPH
.2021.306375.

28. Task Force on Research Specific to Pregnant Women and Lactating
Women, *Report Implementation Plan,* August 2020, https://www.nichd.nih
.gov/sites/default/files/inline-files/PRGLAC_Implement_Plan_083120
.pdf; National Institute of Child Health and Human Development, "Task
Force on Research Specific to Pregnant Women and Lactating Women,"
last updated October 20, 2022, https://www.nichd.nih.gov/about/advisory
/PRGLAC.

29. Endocrine Society, "Hormones and Menopause: What You Need to
Know," accessed July 14, 2023, https://www.endocrine.org/-/media/endo
crine/files/patient-engagement/hormones-and-series/hormones_and
_menopause_what_you_need_to_know.pdf.

30. Saad Samargandy et al., "Arterial Stiffness Accelerates Within 1 Year of the Final Menstrual Period: The SWAN Heart Study," *Arteriosclerosis, Thrombosis, and Vascular Biology* 40, no. 4 (2020): 1001–8, https://doi.org /10.1161/ATVBAHA.119.313622.

31. Opinium Research, *Menopause Research,* Vodafone, October 15, 2021, https://www.vodafone.com/sites/default/files/2021-10/menopause-global -research-report-2021.pdf.

32. Newson Health Menopause Society, "Impact of Perimenopause and Menopause on Work," January 16, 2022, https://www.nhmenopause society.org/research/impact-of-perimenopause-and-menopause-on-work/.

33. Deb Gordon, "73% of Women Don't Treat Their Menopause Symptoms, New Survey Shows," *Forbes,* July 13, 2021, https://www.forbes.com/sites /debgordon/2021/07/13/73-of-women-dont-treat-their-menopause -symptoms-new-survey-shows/?sh=647ec37c454f.

34. Juliana M. Kling et al., "Menopause Management Knowledge in Postgraduate Family Medicine, Internal Medicine, and Obstetrics and Gynecology Residents: A Cross-Sectional Survey," *Mayo Clinic Proceedings* 94, no. 2 (2019): 242–53, https://doi.org/10.1016/j.mayocp.2018.08.033.

35. Michelle M. Mielke, "Effects of Bilateral Oophorectomy on Physical and Cognitive Aging," Mayo Clinic SCORE on Sex Differences, accessed July 14, 2023, https://www.mayo.edu/research/centers-programs/mayo -clinic-score-sex-differences/research-projects/effects-bilateral-oopho rectomy-physical-cognitive-aging.

36. Kejal Katarci and Kent R. Bailey, "Effects of Bilateral Oophorectomy on Imaging Biomarkers of Alzheimer's Disease and Cerebrovascular Diseases," Mayo Clinic SCORE on Sex Differences, accessed July 14, 2023, https://www.mayo.edu/research/centers-programs/mayo-clinic -score-sex-differences/research-projects/bilateral-oophorectomy-imaging -biomarkers-alzheimers-cerebrovascular-diseases.

37. Nathan K. LeBrasseur, "Effects of Bilateral Oophorectomy on the Biology of Physical and Cognitive Aging in a Murine Model," Mayo Clinic SCORE on Sex Differences, accessed July 14, 2023, https://www .mayo.edu/research/centers-programs/mayo-clinic-score-sex-differences /research-projects/effects-ovariectomy-biology-physical-cognitive-aging -mice.

## CHAPTER 10

1. Arthur A. Mirin, "Gender Disparity in the Funding of Diseases by the U.S. National Institutes of Health," *Journal of Women's Health* 30, no. 7 (2021): 956–63, https://www.ncbi.nlm.nih.gov/pmc/articles/PMC 8290307/.

2. Mayo Clinic, "Women's Health Research Center," accessed July 14, 2023, https://www.mayo.edu/research/centers-programs/womens-health -research-center/overview.

3. Autoimmune Association, "Autoimmune Facts," accessed July 14, 2023, https://autoimmune.org/wp-content/uploads/2019/12/1-in-5-Brochure.pdf.

4. Alzheimer's Association, "2023 Alzheimer's Disease Facts and Figures: The Patient Journey in an Era of New Treatments," *Alzheimer's & Dementia* 19, no. 4 (2023), https://doi.org/10.1002/alz.13016.

5. Office on Women's Health, "Urinary Tract Infections," last updated February 22, 2021, https://www.womenshealth.gov/a-z-topics/urinary-tract-infections.

6. International Foundation for Gastrointestinal Disorders, "IBS Facts and Statistics," accessed July 14, 2023, https://aboutibs.org/what-is-ibs/facts-about-ibs/.

7. Shailja C. Shah et al., "Sex-Based Differences in Incidence of Inflammatory Bowel Diseases—Pooled Analysis of Population-Based Studies from Western Countries," *Gastroenterology* 155, no. 4 (2018): 1079–89.e3, https://doi.org/10.1053/j.gastro.2018.06.043.

8. Thomas Greuter et al., on behalf of Swiss IBDnet, an official working group of the Swiss Society of Gastroenterology, "Gender Differences in Inflammatory Bowel Disease," *Digestion* 29, no. 101, suppl. 1 (2020): 98–104, https://doi.org/10.1159/000504701.

9. Neda Sarafrazi, Edwina A. Wambogo and John A. Shepherd, "Osteoporosis or Low Bone Mass in Older Adults: United States, 2017–2018," NCHS Data Brief No. 405, March 2021, https://www.cdc.gov/nchs/products/databriefs/db405.htm.

10. American Thyroid Association, "General Information/Press Room," accessed July 14, 2023, https://www.thyroid.org/media-main/press-room/#:~:text=Prevalence%20and%20Impact%20of%20Thyroid%20Disease&text=Up%20to%2060%20percent%20of,thyroid%20disorder%20during%20her%20lifetime.

11. Autoimmune Association, "What Is Autoimmunity?," accessed October 3, 2023, https://autoimmune.org/resource-center/about-autoimmunity/.

12. Frederick W. Miller, "The Increasing Prevalence of Autoimmunity and Autoimmune Diseases: An Urgent Call to Action for Improved Understanding, Diagnosis, Treatment, and Prevention," *Current Opinion in Immunology* (February 2023): 102266, https://www.sciencedirect.com/science/article/abs/pii/S0952791522001133.

13. Maunil K. Desai and Roberta Diaz Brinton, "Autoimmune Disease in Women: Endocrine Transition and Risk Across the Lifespan," *Frontiers in Endocrinology* 10 (2019), https://doi.org/10.3389/fendo.2019.00265.

14. Autoimmune Association News, "The Autoimmune Association Supports Recommendations of Report to Advance Research for Autoimmune Diseases," Autoimmune Association, June 16, 2022, https://autoimmune.org/autoimmune-association-supports-recommendations-of-reports-to-advance-research-for-autoimmune-diseases/#:~:text=NIH%20is%20the

%20primary%20funding,percent%20between%202013%20and%20
2020.

15. The National Academies of Sciences, Engineering, and Medicine,
"Enhancing NIH Research on Autoimmune Disease: Highlights
Consensus Study," May 2022, https://nap.nationalacademies.org/resource
/26554/Enhancing_NIH_Research_on_Autoimmune_Disease_High
lights.pdf.

16. Autoimmune Association, "The Autoimmune Association Supports
Recommendations of Report to Advance Research for Autoimmune
Diseases."

17. National Institutes of Health, "Office of Autoimmune Disease Research
(OADR-ORWH)," accessed October 3, 2023, https://orwh.od.nih.gov
/OADR-ORWH.

18. Nolan, interview.

19. Landon G. vom Steeg and Sabra L. Klein, "SeXX Matters in Infectious
Disease Pathogenesis," *PLoS Pathogens* 12, no. 2 (2016): e1005374, https://
doi.org/10.1371/journal.ppat.1005374.

20. Sabra L. Klein and Andrew Pekosz, "Sex-Based Biology and the Rational
Design of Influenza Vaccination Strategies," *Journal of Infectious Diseases*
209, suppl. 3 (2014): S114–9, https://doi.org/10.1093/infdis/jiu066.

21. Samer A. Kharroubi and Marwa Diab-El-Harake, "Sex-Differences in
COVID-19 Diagnosis, Risk Factors and Disease Comorbidities: A Large
US-Based Cohort Study," *Frontiers in Public Health* 10 (2022), https://doi
.org/10.3389/fpubh.2022.1029190.

22. Talal Ansari and Jennifer Calfas, "Men Died from Covid-19 at Much
Higher Rate Than Women in Pandemic's First Year, " *Wall Street Journal,*
October 25, 2022, https://www.wsj.com/articles/men-died-from-covid-19
-at-much-higher-rate-than-women-during the-first-year-of-pandemic
-11666662323.

23. Shirley V. Sylvester et al., "Sex Differences in Sequelae from COVID-19
Infection and in Long COVID Syndrome: A Review," *Current Medical
Research and Opinion* 38, no. 8 (2022): 1391–99, https://doi.org/10.1080
/03007995.2022.2081454.

24. National Institute of Child Health and Human Development, "Do Some
Babies Have a Higher Risk of Severe COVID-19?," February 7, 2022,
https://covid19.nih.gov/news-and-stories/do-some-babies-have-higher-risk
-severe-covid-19#:~:text=Pregnant%20people%20who%20recovered%20
from,to%20transfer%20to%20male%20fetuses.

25. Janna R. Shapiro et al., "Association of Frailty, Age, and Biological Sex
with Severe Acute Respiratory Syndrome Coronavirus 2 Messenger RNA
Vaccine-Induced Immunity in Older Adults," *Clinical Infectious Diseases:
An Official Publication of the Infectious Diseases Society of America* 75, suppl.
1 (2022): S61–71, https://doi.org/10.1093/cid/ciac397; Janna R. Shapiro
et al., "Sex-Specific Effects of Aging on Humoral Immune Responses to

Repeated Influenza Vaccination in Older Adults," *NPJ Vaccines* 6, no. 1 (2021): 147, https://doi.org/10.1038/s41541-021-00412-6.

26. Donald F. Weaver, "Alzheimer's Disease as an Innate Autoimmune Disease (AD$^2$): A New Molecular Paradigm," *Alzheimer's & Dementia,* first published September 27, 2022, https://alz-journals.onlinelibrary.wiley.com /doi/full/10.1002/alz.12789#:~:text=In%20the%20AD2%20model%2C %20AD%20is%20a%20brain%2Dcentric,larger%2C%20comprehensive %20conceptualization%20of%20AD.

27. Sarah C. Janicki and Nicole Schupf, "Hormonal Influences on Cognition and Risk for Alzheimer Disease," *Current Neurology and Neuroscience Reports,* September 2010, https://www.ncbi.nlm.nih.gov/pmc/articles /PMC3058507/#:~:text=Multiple%20lines%20of%20evidence%20 suggest,cognitive%20declines%20associated%20with%20AD.

28. Alzheimer's Association, "2023 Alzheimer's Disease Facts and Figures," special report, accessed October 3, 2023, https://www.alz.org/media /Documents/alzheimers-facts-and-figures.pdf.

29. Ibid.

30. Ibid.

31. Andrew E. Budson, "Why Are Women More Likely to Develop Alzheimer's Disease?," Harvard Health Publishing, January 20, 2022, https://www.health.harvard.edu/blog/why-are-women-more-likely-to -develop-alzheimers-disease-202201202672; David Kang and Alexa Woo, "Why Women May Be More Susceptible to Alzheimer's Disease," NewsWise, October 4, 2022, https://www.newswise.com/articles/why -women-may-be-more-susceptible-to-alzheimer-s-disease?sc=mwhr&xy =10023932.

32. Alzheimer's Association, "2023 Alzheimer's Disease Facts and Figures."

33. Ibid.

34. HealthyWomen, "Alzheimer's Disease," accessed October 3, 2023, https:// www.healthywomen.org/condition/alzheimers-disease-hub/.

35. HealthyWomen editors, "You and Your Brain: A Collaboration of HealthyWomen, Prevention and Women's Alzheimer's Movement at Cleveland Clinic," December 6, 2022, https://www.healthywomen.org /programs/your-brain-prevention-alzheimers-movement.

36. FDA Drug Trial Snapshots, October 4, 2023, https://www.fda.gov/drugs /drug-approvals-and-databases/drug-trials-snapshots.

37. Myreen E. Tomas et al., "Overdiagnosis of Urinary Tract Infection and Underdiagnosis of Sexually Transmitted Infection in Adult Women Presenting to an Emergency Department," *Journal of Clinical Microbiology* 53, no. 8 (2015): 2686–92, https://doi.org/10.1128/JCM.00670-15.

38. Tamara Bhandari, "Recurrent UTIs Linked to Gut Microbiome, Chronic Inflammation," Washington University School of Medicine in St. Louis, May 2, 2022, https://medicine.wustl.edu/news/recurrent-utis-linked-to -gut-microbiome-chronic-inflammation/.

39. Ibid.
40. International Foundation for Gastrointestinal Disorders, "IBS Facts and Statistics," accessed September 9, 2023, https://aboutibs.org/what-is-ibs /facts-about-ibs/.
41. "Irritable Bowel Syndrome Patients Suffer High Rates of Anxiety and Depression," University of Missouri School of Medicine, February 22, 2023, https://medicine.missouri.edu/news/irritable-bowel-syndrome -patients-suffer-high-rates-anxiety-and-depression.
42. International Foundation for Gastrointestinal Disorders, "IBS in Women," accessed July 17, 2023, https://aboutibs.org/what-is-ibs/ibs-in-women/; Yong Sung Kim et al., "Sex Differences in Gut Microbiota," *World Journal of Men's Health* 38, no. 1 (2020): 48–60, https://doi.org/10.5534/wjmh .190009.
43. Ibid.
44. Zahid Ijaz Tarar et al., "Burden of Anxiety and Depression Among Hospitalized Patients with Irritable Bowel Syndrome: A Nationwide Analysis," *Irish Journal of Medical Science* 192, no. 5 (October 2023): 2159–66, https://pubmed.ncbi.nlm.nih.gov/36593438/.
45. Neuroscience News, "Irritable Bowel Syndrome Patients May Suffer Significantly Higher Rates of Anxiety, Depression and Suicidal Ideation," February 22, 2023, https://neurosciencenews.com/ibs-mental-health -22548/.
46. Ashley Bell, "Symptoms of IBS in Women vs. Men," UCLA David Geffen School of Medicine, April 19, 2023, https://medschool.ucla.edu/news -article/symptoms-of-ibs-in-women-vs-men.
47. Thomas Greuter et al., "Gender Differences in Inflammatory Bowel Disease," *Digestion* 101, Suppl. 1 (January 29, 2020): 98–104, https://doi .org/10.1159/000504701.
48. Karen Nitkin, "Crohn's and Ulcerative Colitis Pose Special Concerns for Women," Johns Hopkins Medicine News and Publications, May 11, 2020, https://www.hopkinsmedicine.org/news/articles/2020/05/crohns-and -ulcerative-colitis-pose-special-concerns-for-women#:~:text=Women%20 with%20IBD%20are%20also,fetus%20will%20experience%20side%20 effects.
49. Woods's story is abridged, with permission, from Renika Woods, "After Years of Suffering and Shame, I Am Now a Proud Crohn's Warrior," HealthyWomen, April 22, 2021, https://military.healthywomen.org /after-years-of-suffering-and-shame-im-now-a-proud-crohns-warrior/.
50. Tabby Khan et al., "Women with Inflammatory Bowel Disease Wait Longer for Diagnosis and Treatment, Despite Presenting Earlier with Red-Flag Symptoms," Komodo Health, May 10, 2022, https://www .komodohealth.com/insights/women-inflammatory-bowel-disease.
51. Laura Sempere et al., "Gender Biases and Diagnostic Delay in Inflammatory Bowel Disease: Multicenter Observational Study,"

*Inflammatory Bowel Diseases,* January 31, 2023, https://doi.org/10.1093
/ibd/izad001.

52. Bone Health and Osteoporosis Foundation, "13 Leading Aging, Caregiver
and Women's Health Groups Join Forces to Reduce Common and Costly
Bone Fractures," May 29, 2019, https://www.bonehealthandosteoporosis
.org/news/13-leading-aging-caregiver-and-womens-health-groups-join
-forces-to-reduce-common-and-costly-bone-fractures/.
53. Michele F. Bellantoni, "Osteoporosis Information," Johns Hopkins
Arthritis Center, accessed October 3, 2023, https://www.hopkinsarthritis
.org/arthritis-info/osteoporosis-info/#:~:text=How%20common%20is%20
osteoporosis%3F,bone%20mass%20increases%20with%20age.
54. Mark Richens, "10 Things to Know About Racial Differences in Bone
Health," American Bone Health, April 13, 2020, https://americanbone
health.org/races-ethnicities/10-things-to-know-about-racial-differences-in
-bone-health/.
55. Stephen K. Liu et al., "Quality of Osteoporosis Care of Older Medicare
Recipients with Fragility Fractures: 2006 to 2010," *Journal of the American
Geriatrics Society* 61, no. 11 (2013): 1855–62, https://doi.org/10.1111/jgs
.12507.
56. Jeffrey R. Curtis et al., "Population-Based Fracture Risk Assessment and
Osteoporosis Treatment Disparities by Race and Gender," *Journal of
General Internal Medicine* 24, no. 8 (2009): 956–62, https://doi.org/10
.1007/s11606-009-1031-8.
57. Bellantoni, "Osteoporosis Information."
58. Shouts's story is abridged, with permission, from Cecilia Shouts, "It
Wasn't Muscle Damage: It Was Four Fractures and Osteoporosis,"
HealthyWomen, October 20, 2021, https://www.healthywomen.org
/created-with-support/it-was-four-fractures-osteoporosis.
59. Jennifer S. R. Mammen and Anne R. Cappola, "Autoimmune Thyroid
Disease in Women," *JAMA* 325, no. 23 (2021): 2392, https://doi.org/10
.1001/jama.2020.22196.
60. Elizabeth A. McAninch, Jennifer S. Glueck and Antonio C. Bianco, "Does
Sex Bias Play a Role for Dissatisfied Patients with Hypothyroidism?,"
*Journal of the Endocrine Society* 2, no. 8 (2018): 970–73, https://doi.org
/10.1210/js.2018-00169.
61. "Therapeutics," *Journal of the American Medical Association,* 1910, quoted
in McAninch, Glueck and Bianco, "Does Sex Bias Play a Role for
Dissatisfied Patients with Hypothyroidism?"
62. Ibid.
63. Mammen and Cappola, "Autoimmune Thyroid Disease in Women."
64. PhRMA, "Medicines in Development 2022 Report: Chronic Diseases,"
September 29, 2022, https://phrma.org/en/resource-center/Topics
/Medicines-in-Development/Medicines-in-Development-for-Chronic
-Diseases-2022-Report.

65. The National Breast Cancer Foundation, "Breast Cancer Facts & Stats," accessed September 9, 2023, https://www.nationalbreastcancer.org/breast -cancer-facts/#:~:text=Breast%20cancer%20in%20men%20statistics &text=Although%20rare%2C%20men%20get%20breast,cancer%20 in%20the%20United%20States.&text=An%20estimated%20530%20 U.S.%20men%20will%20die%20from%20breast%20cancer%20in%20 2023.&text=The%20lifetime%20risk%20of%20a,is%20about%201%20 in%20833.
66. Ibid.

## CHAPTER 11

1. Wikipedia, "Medical Device Regulation Act," last updated May 5, 2023, https://en.wikipedia.org/wiki/Medical_Device_Regulation_Act#:~:text =The%20U.S.%20legislation%20enacted%20in,Roosevelt; Ford Presidential Library, White House Records Office: Legislation Case Files, Ann Arbor, MI, Records of the Medical Device Amendments of 1976, box 45, folder 5/28/76 S510; https://www.fordlibrarymuseum.gov/library /document/0055/1669327.pdf.
2. Food and Drug Administration, "Evaluation of Sex-Specific Data in Medical Device Clinical Studies: Guidance for Industry and Food and Drug Administration Staff," August 22, 2014, https://www.fda.gov /regulatory-information/search-fda-guidance-documents/evaluation-sex -specific-data-medical-device-clinical-studies-guidance-industry-and-food -and-drug.
3. Marina Walker Guevara, "We Used AI to Identify the Sex of 340,000 People Harmed by Medical Devices," International Consortium of Investigative Journalists, November 25, 2019, https://www.icij.org /investigations/implant-files/we-used-ai-to-identify-the-sex-of-340000 -people-harmed-by-medical-devices/.
4. Susan P. Phillips, Katrina Gee and Laura Wells, "Medical Devices, Invisible Women, Harmful Consequences," *International Journal of Environmental Research and Public Health* 19, no. 21 (2022): 14524, https:// doi.org/10.3390/ijerph192114524.
5. Hamid Ghanbari et al., "Effectiveness of Implantable Cardioverter-Defibrillators for the Primary Prevention of Sudden Cardiac Death in Women with Advanced Heart Failure: A Meta-Analysis of Randomized Controlled Trials," *Archives of Internal Medicine* 169, no. 16 (September 14, 2009): 1500–6, https://pubmed.ncbi.nlm.nih.gov/19752408/.
6. US Food and Drug Administration, "Concerns About Metal-on-Metal Hip Implants," last updated March 15, 2019, https://www.fda.gov/medical -devices/metal-metal-hip-implants/concerns-about-metal-metal-hip -implants.
7. Bryan D. Haughom et al., "Do Complication Rates Differ by Gender After Metal-on-Metal Hip Resurfacing Arthroplasty? A Systematic Review,"

*Clinical Orthopaedics and Related Research* 473, no. 8 (August 2015): 2521–29, https://www.ncbi.nlm.nih.gov/pmc/articles/PMC4488218/.

8. Sophie N. Putka, "Hips That Harm: When Medical Devices Fail Women," CUNY Academic Works, December 18, 2020, https://academic works.cuny.edu/cgi/viewcontent.cgi?article=1478&context=gj_etds; Maria C. S. Inacio et al., "Sex and Risk of Hip Implant Failure," *JAMA Internal Medicine* 173, no. 6 (2013): 435, https://doi.org/10.1001/jamainternmed .2013.3271.

9. US Food and Drug Administration, "Metal-on-Metal Hip Implants," last updated September 30, 2019, https://www.fda.gov/medical-devices /implants-and-prosthetics/metal-metal-hip-implants.

10. Madris Kinard and Rita F. Redberg, "Is the FDA Failing Women?," *AMA Journal of Ethics* 23, no. 9 (2021): E750–56, https://journalofethics.ama -assn.org/article/fda-failing-women/2021-09.

11. FDA Center for Devices and Radiological Health, "Health of Women Strategic Plan," January 2022, https://www.fda.gov/media/155461/down load?attachment.

## CODA: HIGHLIGHTS FROM 2000 THROUGH 2023

1. Organization for the Study of Sex Differences, "History of the OSSD," accessed July 17, 2023, https://www.ossdweb.org/history; Institute of Medicine (US) Committee on Understanding the Biology of Sex and Gender Differences, *Exploring the Biological Contributions to Human Health: Does Sex Matter?*, edited by T. M. Wizemann and M. L. Pardue (Washington, DC: National Academies Press, 2001), https://www.ncbi .nlm.nih.gov/books/NBK222288/.

2. Institute of Medicine (US) Committee on Understanding and Eliminating Racial and Ethnic Disparities in Health Care, *Unequal Treatment, Confronting Racial and Ethnic Disparities in Health Care,* edited by Brian D. Smedley, Adrienne Y. Stith and Alan R. Nelson (Washington, DC: National Academies Press, 2003), https://www.ncbi.nlm.nih.gov/books /NBK220358/.

3. Women's Health Office Act of 2009, H.R.3242, 111th Congress (2009–2010), https://www.congress.gov/bill/111th-congress/house-bill/3242 ?s=1&r=94.

4. *Biology of Sex Differences,* published by BMC, part of Springer Nature, https://bsd.biomedcentral.com/.

5. The Society for Women's Health Research and US Food and Drug Administration Office of Women's Health, *Dialogues on Diversifying Clinical Trials: Successful Strategies for Engaging Women and Minorities in Clinical Trials,* September 22–23, 2011, Washington, DC, https:// www.fda.gov/files/science%20&%20research/published/White -Paper-on-the-Dialogues-on-Diversifying-Clinical-Trials-Conference .pdf.

6. NIH Office of Research on Women's Health, "2019–2023 Trans-NIH Strategic Plan for Women's Health Research," presentation on the plan took place at the 46th Meeting of the Advisory Committee on Research on Women's Health in October 2018, https://orwh.od.nih.gov/about/trans -nih-strategic-plan-womens-health-research.

7. Office of Research on Women's Health, National Institutes of Health, and US Department of Health and Human Services, "Moving into the Future with New Dimensions and Strategies: A Vision for 2020 for Women's Health Research: Strategic Plan," accessed October 3, 2023, https://orwh. od.nih.gov/sites/orwh/files/docs/ORWH_StrategicPlan2020 _Vol1.pdf.

8. Ning Ding et al., "Per- and Polyfluoroalkyl Substances and Incident Hypertension in Multi-Racial/Ethnic Women: The Study of Women's Health Across the Nation," *Hypertension* 79, no. 8 (August 2022): 1876– 86, https://www.ahajournals.org/doi/10.1161/HYPERTENSIONAHA .121.18809.

9. Michelle Long et al., "Women's Experiences with Provider Communication and Interactions in Health Care Settings: Findings from the 2022 KFF Women's Health Survey," Kaiser Family Foundation, February 22, 2023, https://www.kff.org/womens-health-policy/issue-brief /womens-experiences-with-provider-communication-interactions-health -care-settings-findings-from-2022-kff-womens-health-survey/.

### CHAPTER 12

1. Michelle Long et al., "Women's Experiences with Provider Communication and Interactions in Health Care Settings: Findings from the 2022 KFF Women's Health Survey," Kaiser Family Foundation, February 22, 2023, https://www.kff.org/womens-health-policy/issue-brief /womens-experiences-with-provider-communication-interactions-health -care-settings-findings-from-2022-kff-womens-health-survey/.

# INDEX

264    Index